X

18.4.08

The Informed Practice Nurse

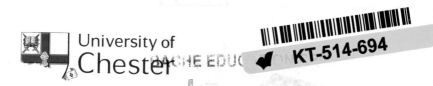

The Informed Practice Nurse

Second Edition

Edited by Marilyn Edwards

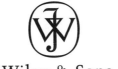

John Wiley & Sons, Ltd

Other Wiley Editorial Offices

John Wiley & Sons Inc., 111 River Street, Hoboken, NJ 07030, USA

Jossey-Bass, 989 Market Street, San Francisco, CA 94103-1741, USA

Wiley-VCH Verlag GmbH, Boschstr. 12, D-69469 Weinheim, Germany

John Wiley & Sons Australia Ltd, 42 McDougall Street, Milton, Queensland 4064, Australia

John Wiley & Sons (Asia) Pte Ltd, 2 Clementi Loop #02-01, Jin Xing Distripark, Singapore
129809

John Wiley & Sons Canada Ltd, 6045 Freemont Blvd, Mississauga, ONT, L5R 4J3, Canada

Wiley also publishes its books in a variety of electronic formats. Some content that appears in
print may not be available in electronic books.

Library of Congress Cataloging-in-Publication Data

The informed practice nurse / edited by Marilyn Edwards. – 2nd ed.
  p. ; cm.
  Includes bibliographical references and index.
  ISBN 978-0-470-05749-0 (pbk. : alk. paper)
1. Nurse practitioners–Great Britain.   2. Primary care (Medicine)–Great Britain.
I. Edwards, Marilyn.
  [DNLM: 1. Nursing Care–methods–Great Britain.   2. Family Practice–
Great Britain.   3. Nurse Practitioners–Great Britain.   4. Nursing Process–Great Britain.
WY 100 I43 2007]
  RT82.8.I53 2007
  610.7306′92–dc22

                                                              2007029988

A catalogue record for this book is available from the British Library

ISBN: 978-0-470-05749-0

Typeset by SNP Best-set Typesetter Ltd., Hong Kong
Printed and bound in Singapore by Markono Print Media Pte Ltd
This book is printed on acid-free paper responsibly manufactured from sustainable forestry
in which at least two trees are planted for each one used for paper production.

This book is dedicated to my husband Chris who has encouraged and supported me in developing from a novice Practice Nurse to an Advanced Nurse Practitioner.

Contents

Contributors

Chris Baldwin RGN, School Nurse Cert, FP Cert, Dip Infection Prevention and Control. Clinical Nurse Specialist Infection Control, North Staffordshire Primary Care Trust

Mandy Beaumont MPH, RGN, Cert Infection Control Nursing. Health Protection Nurse, Health Protection Agency, West Midlands North, Health Protection Unit

Marilyn Edwards MSc, BSc(Hons) SRN, FEATC, FPCert. Advanced Nurse Practitioner, Bilbrook Medical Centre, Bilbrook, Staffordshire

Diana Forster MSC, BA(Hons), RGN, RM, RHV, RHVT, RNT. Formerly Head of Health Studies, University of North London

Susan Jones BSc, SRD. Paediatric Dietician, New Cross Hospital, Wolverhampton

Gudrun Limbrick BA(Hons). Freelance writer, founder of Lesbian Health Group, LesBeWell

Karen Mayne RGN, OHND, BSc(Hons), Dip Advanced Nursing Practice (Primary Care). Nurse Practitioner, Moorfield House Surgery, Hereford

Cath Molineux MSc, BSc(Hons), OND, OHNC. Specialist Practitioner in General Practice at time of writing first edition

Georgina Paget BSc(Hons), RGN, OND(Hons). Clinical Nurse Specialist in HIV/AIDS for First Community Health NHS Trust, South Staffordshire

Diane Pannell SRN, SCM, DipMid, HECert. Formerly Community Midwife, Bromsgrove and Redditch

Wendy Okoye RGN, DipPSN(CHN), FP Cert. Team leader, Practice Nurse, Willington Surgery Derby

Joy Rudge MSc, BSc, DipSN, RGN, DN. Tissue Viability Nurse, Wolverhampton PCT

Glen Turp RGN. Royal College of Nursing Regional Officer at time of writing first edition

Pat Tweed MSc, BSc(Hons), SRN, FEATC, FPCert. Specialist Practitioner in General Practice

Preface

The second edition of *The Informed Practice Nurse* has been written in response to the dynamic nature of general practice nursing. Updates from the first edition include reference to Nursing and Midwifery Council and deleting drugs, treatments or managements that are no longer available or recommended. All chapters have been updated with references to reflect topical issues relating to each subject. New material has focused on change management, which recognises the valuable input of practice nurses in their organisations, domestic abuse that affects all strata of society, issues relating to diet and childhood obesity, advances in wound management and the changing role of the practice nurse.

Nurses have to be informed in order to deliver sensitive and holistic care. I hope that each reader will learn at least one new fact that will improve their knowledge and understanding, reflect on it and use it to improve patient care or safety.

Introduction

This book has been planned to meet the needs of practice nurses, and includes many issues that relate to other community nurses and medical colleagues. Examples of real or hypothesised practice, with recommendations for implementing quality care, relate specifically to general practice. The reader can probably refer to other examples to fit particular fields. Most of the chapters are subdivided into specific subject areas. For example, the chapter on Women's Health is subdivided to include the health needs of lesbian women, premenstrual syndrome and domestic violence (domestic abuse). This structuring allows ease of access to these topics.

Nursing ethics underpins all patient care and nursing action, and is essential to protect both nurse and patients (Chapter 1). Personal and professional accountability and patient autonomy, which are integral to all aspects of patient care, are stressed throughout the book and should stay in the forefront of the reader's mind. Most of the chapters interrelate, with topics such as ethics, management and health promotion being essential components of all basic consultations in general practice.

Although the book is not a clinical handbook, wound management (Chapter 8) is included to demonstrate how the introductory chapters relate to patient care. These issues can be transferred to other areas of practice. For example, risk management, informed consent, time management, infection control and health promotion (Chapters 1–4) should be considered for all routine procedures, including child vaccinations and cervical cytology. Health profiling and needs assessment (Chapter 4) is essential when planning a strategy for commissioning and delivering services for men, women and children (Chapters 5–7). Issues relating to domestic abuse relate to all ages and genders.

The practice nurse role continues to develop and expand, with increasing autonomy, skill mix and opportunities for nurse-led clinics. The benefits and drawbacks to these roles are discussed in Chapter 9.

Evidence-based information is crucial to support nursing practice and will be found throughout the text. Inevitably there is some overlap between chapters because topics cannot be compartmentalised. This overlap will reinforce relevant issues. The content of the chapters are explained through a brief précis of the rationale for, and content of, the text. Recommended reading and resource lists, found at the end of each chapter, will assist the reader to access more detailed information on topics that interest them.

It is hoped that issues raised in this book will encourage nurses at all levels to question both own their practice, and that of their medical and nursing colleagues where necessary, and to use evidence-based knowledge to negotiate appropriate care for their patients.

Quality nursing is independent of the political climate with its constant change of health policy; any mention of specific health policy is purely accidental.

Chapter 1

Ethics

Pat Tweed, Cath Molineux and Marilyn Edwards

'Ethics' is derived from the Greek word *ethos*, meaning spirit of a community; this is the collective belief and value system of any moral community, social or professional group (Reeves & Orford 2002). Morals and values are inter-related and integral to society. The study of ethics helps one to consider what kind of things are good or bad and how to decide whether actions are right or wrong. Ethics and the law are closely interwoven, as our laws are usually based on ethics (Holland 2004).

The role of codes of practice in ethical decision making is discussed in this chapter using examples from general practice. The reader will recognise many of the examples cited in the chapter, and will probably be able to describe many more.

In order to assess the effectiveness of codes of practice in making ethical decisions in nursing, one must first consider what is meant by an ethical decision. This chapter examines the codes of practice for nurses, following a brief description of ethical principles. *The Code of Professional Conduct* (Nursing and Midwifery Council 2004) will be referred to as 'the Code', the principles of which may conflict with issues relating to power and authority in the primary healthcare setting. The Code has been reviewed and mod-ernised, and is expected to be rolled out in January 2008 (Nursing and Midwifery Council 2007), but the main principles are unlikely to change.

Doctors and nurses may sometimes forget the rights of patients in the rush to 'get the job done', meet targets and appear efficient. This is an area that nurses can readily address and possibly share with their primary healthcare team colleagues. Informed consent, for both adults and minors, is essential if the patient is to be involved in their care and be autonomous. Patients with a learning disability pose a greater challenge in obtaining informed consent. The issues discussed within this chapter are pertinent to all areas of nursing care, and are referred to throughout the book. There is inevitably some overlap between sections, but this serves to emphasis the importance of certain issues.

The reader is directed to Beauchamp and Childress (2001) for an in-depth discussion on ethical theory.

The Informed Practice Nurse, Edwards, M. (2008), Chichester: Wiley.

For convenience the term 'patient' will be used in the text, although it is recognised that many people who consult the nurses are 'well people'.

Ethics, philosophies and codes of practice

Ethical philosophies and theories

The two main philosophies of ethical reasoning, utilitarianism and deontology, have almost diametrically opposed prime principles (Seedhouse 1998). John Stuart Mill and Jeremy Bentham propounded utilitarianism, believing that the ends justify the means and that the right action is the one that offers the greatest good to the greatest number.

Deontology (derived from the Greek word *deon*, meaning 'duty') is the theory associated with Immanuel Kant. It is based on duty and respect for the individual, who must be treated as an end in themselves and never as a means to an end. It is the action itself that is right or wrong; the consequences are less important.

When faced with a moral dilemma where there are two alternative choices, neither of which seems a satisfactory solution to the problem, a decision has to be made based on one's own moral principles and what each person believes to be right. The rules that guide thinking are known as ethical principles. The four principles of biomedical ethics listed below are discussed in depth by Beauchamp and Childress (2001).

> Autonomy relates to respecting and preserving people's ability to decide for themselves.
> Beneficence is the obligation to provide benefits and balance benefit against risk.
> Non-maleficence refers to the obligation to avoid doing harm.
> Justice is fairness in the distribution of benefits and risks.

In his text on ethical theory and practice, Thiroux (1980) outlines five ethical principles that he considers to be applicable to all spheres of life, adding honesty to the main four principles (Box 1.1).

Box 1.1   Ethical principles, applicable to all spheres of life (Thiroux 1980)

- The value of life and respect for persons
- Goodness or rightness
- Justice or fairness
- Truth telling or honesty
- Individual freedom or autonomy

The functions of codes of practice

The three functions of professional codes identified by Burnard and Chapman (1988) are ethical, political and disciplinary. This section will concentrate mainly on the first of these, although the impact of the other two will be clearly shown. Codes of practice are recommended by professional organisations, as many types of human conduct are harmful, although not illegal (Seedhouse 1998).

Codes of practice are meant to inform and reassure members of the public about the quality of the professional service, as well as enhancing the public image of the individual practitioner. The purpose of the code is to inform the profession of the standard of professional conduct required of them in the exercise of their professional accountability and practice (Nursing and Midwifery Council 2004). It can be used to fight for improvements in standards, although this is not always an easy path to take, as will be seen later.

Professional codes also play a part in supporting the status of a profession. A code of conduct has been said to be one of the defining characteristics of a profession (Jaggar, quoted in Chadwick & Tadd 1992). The implication is that those within the group can be trusted to regulate their members and, if necessary, to discipline them if they fail to uphold the high standards of the code.

However, the Nursing and Midwifery Council (NMC) Code of Professional Conduct is issued for guidance and advice, laying a moral responsibility rather than a statutory duty on members of the profession (Young 1989). The Code can be used by a nurse to measure her own conduct, in the knowledge that the requirements of the Code are used by the NMC during trials of misconduct. Failure to comply with the Code may result in a nurse losing her registration. The Code of Professional Conduct is therefore a guide, a political statement and a means of regulating the profession.

The emphasis of the Code

The NMC Code sets out the professional accountability of each registered nurse, midwife and health visitor working in clinical and management settings. Although the Code may have considerable influence over a nurse's resolution of ethical dilemmas, each situation for each person is unique, and is only a guide to decision making. A code may stress the most important considerations that should influence a decision, but a nurse cannot turn to the Code and expect it to provide a moral answer to an ethical problem Nurses do not leave their moral choices behind when they are at work (Chadwick & Tadd 1992).

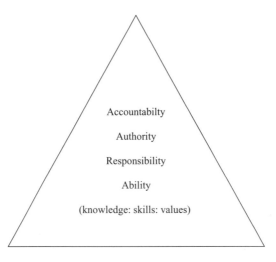

Figure 1.1   Preconditions to accountability (from Bergman 1981).

The Code commits each individual nurse, midwife and health visitor to safeguard and promote the interests of both society and individual patients. It also requires that each shall act in such a way that justifies the trust and confidence of the public, and uphold and enhance the good reputation of the professions. In order for the nurse to fulfil these requirements, emphasis is placed on four main areas: knowledge, skill, responsibility and accountability; these were the basis of the principles of the Scope of Professional Practice (United Kingdom Central Council for Nursing, Midwifery and Health Visiting (UKCC) 1992).

Bergman (1981) listed four preconditions to accountability, which were almost the same as the areas defined by the Code, but also included the need for authority (Figure 1.1).

Knowledge and skill

The Code places on the practitioner the continuing responsibility to maintain and develop their knowledge, skill and competence, through self-assessment and the production of a personal portfolio. Clause 6 clearly states that each nurse must acknowledge personal limits of knowledge and skill and take steps to remedy any relevant deficits in order to meet the needs of patients; a reflection of Thiroux's principle of honesty.

The Code does not say what each nurse must learn, but acts as a guide. A nurse, faced with the dilemma of being asked or instructed to carry out a procedure that they do not feel fully competent to do has the support of clear principles on which to act.

The perception of competence can differ between a nurse and the employer (Jones 1996, p.83). This is a common situation in general practice, where the old medical adage of 'see one, do one, teach one' is often quoted. The ethical principles involved here are non-maleficence, the primacy of the patients' interest (respect for persons) and the justification of public trust. Castledine (1992) stressed that an individual nurse should feel safe and secure in their own performance before undertaking any task.

Responsibility and accountability

Responsibility and accountability are closely linked, but not synonymous. Accountability is the acceptance of that responsibility, the willingness to explain one's actions and to receive credit or blame for the results of those actions (Evans 1993). One can be responsible but not accountable, though one cannot be accountable without being responsible (Young 1989). A registered nurse, midwife or health visitor is accountable to the patient, the profession, the law and the employer. This is shown in Figure 1.2, which indicates the groups to whom the registered nurse is accountable, the basis of that accountability and the authority empowered to judge the actions of the nurse in each area.

Practice nurses are developing their role in primary healthcare, often by taking over work that was previously seen as the province of the doctor. This role should develop in response to patient need and through experience gained by post-basic education. In general practice, this development has

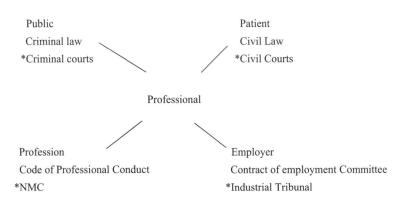

Figure 1.2 Areas of professional accountability.
*represents the authority empowered to judge the actions of the nurse in each area.

resulted in nurses taking the lead in the management of chronic conditions such as asthma, diabetes and coronary heart disease. The role requires both medical knowledge and nursing skills of education, health promotion and counselling. Patients should be included in all the stages of decision making in their care, thus protecting patient autonomy (Clause 2 of the Code). However, it is all too easy to take on the medical model of treatment and cure, accepting delegation of a task, such as the application of cryocautery, from a doctor (Jones 1996, p 125). Nursing skills can be soon forgotten in the excitement and interest of new technology. Nurses who develop assessment and prescribing skills will be aware of their competencies and accountability.

The degree of accountability within a particular situation must surely be linked to the measure of authority held by the individual, as without that authority, one is not free to make an ethical decision regarding a problem (Tadd 1994). The Code does not mention this concept in relation to accountability, but insists that all practitioners are equally accountable.

Issues of power and authority

In a work situation, conflict may arise between the humanist values of the Code and the authoritarian values of the organisation. Safeguarding and promoting the interests of patients and patients may or may not mean following instructions (Tschudin 1994a).

Challenging action could be considered as advocacy on behalf of a patient. An advocate is one who pleads on behalf of another, influencing those who have power for those without (Reeves & Orford 2002). This is a positive, constructive activity recommended as a role for nursing by the UKCC (1989), particularly where a person is incapable of giving informed consent. The Code, Clause 2.4, includes helping individuals access health and social care, information and support relevant to their needs. The issue of informed consent will be addressed later in this chapter.

The nurse–doctor relationship

Traditionally the doctors made all decisions regarding the care of the patients, and imposed their authority over the work or decisions of other members of the team; work in which they had no particular training or skill. Modern practice has fortunately changed this relationship to one of complementary respect for roles. Chadwick and Tadd (1992) argue that where issues are of an ethical nature, the doctor has no particular expertise and should not hold power. The nurse has a responsibility to point out poor practice, to explain current thinking and, if necessary, refuse to take part in a procedure;

refusing, for example, to assist in minor surgery with unsterile instruments (see Chapter 3), or to apply a dressing that could prejudice wound healing and may cause harm (see Chapter 8).

The doctor's authority in medical matters is only legitimate if they perform correctly. The nurse must intervene if they know or suspect it to be wrong (Chadwick & Tadd 1992). In acting to safeguard the well-being of a patient (Clause 1), the nurse must be aware that although this may mean acting as the patient's advocate, they must not place themselves outside other sections of the law by refusing to co-operate with treatment that the doctor has prescribed (Young 1989, p 206).

If the problem were of a serious nature the nurse may feel it necessary, in order to protect the patient (Clause 8), to report the matter to a higher authority. This may be an informal discussion with the head of the clinical governance committee at the Primary Care Trust, if the nurse does not have a nurse manager. The probable harm, in the form of damage to team relationships, or public mistrust, should it become more widely known, must be weighed against the benefit to patient care. This has been demonstrated by the ability of Harold Shipman to cover his malpractice for so long. No one likes to make a fuss, but nurses have a responsibility to share their concerns.

Truth and trust

Trust has to be earned; it places obligations on the individual nurse, not the least of which is honesty. Clause 3.1 includes the need for information to be accurate and truthful, although Reeves and Orford (2002) raise the issue of being economical with the truth, or telling white lies. Failure to be honest with a patient and answer questions relating, for example, to an incurable disease, because of a moral decision made by medical staff and/or relatives, conflicts with obligations relating to competency, consent and right to information. This is likely to destroy the relationship of trust and confidence. The responsibility to provide information rests with the practitioner and 'if something less than the whole truth is told, it should never be because the practitioner is unable to cope with the effects of telling the truth' (UKCC 1989).

Abuse of the individual practitioner

Nurses have always accepted the need to do their best under difficult circumstances, even to the extent of pretending they can cope, when they clearly cannot (Pyne 1994). Clause 8.4 states that the nurse's first consideration in all activities must be the interests and safety of the patient. Nursing management has a responsibility to draw attention to inadequacy of resources when an unacceptable workload is placed on individual practitioners (Clause 8.3).

Pyne (1992) urged nurses to support each other in the interests of the patient, but many practice nurses still work alone, so that the need for a system of peer support, with a route to senior nurses within the health authority is vital. Practice nurse forums and clinical supervision are two means of offering and sharing support (see Chapter 9). They can provide guidance to help address a problem, as peers may have dealt with similar scenarios.

The ethical principle of respect for persons applies to colleagues as well as to patients (Tschudin 1994b). Despite Clause 8.3, nurses will still feel vulnerable if they complain about colleagues, although less so if complaining about working conditions or equipment.

Confidentiality

Confidentiality, in the clinical setting, implies respect for information about a patient that has been given in trust. This information will not be passed to other people without the consent of the patient, except where disclosure is required by law, or by the order of a court, or is necessary in the public interest (Clause 5). Breaches of confidentiality should be regarded as exceptional. Clause 5.1 states that the nurse should ensure that patients understand that some information may be made available to other members of the team involved in the delivery of care. Patient-held records involve the patient sharing in, and having ownership of, his own record. Diabetes, rheumatoid arthritis and ante-natal are examples of conditions where records may be shared by a variety of professionals, but the patient must be a partner in this, controlling the flow of information and not just transporting the card.

On occasions a patient may share personal information that they do not want recorded or passed to a third person. They have a right to expect that their wishes will be complied with, for if they cannot rely on respect for confidences, they will be unlikely to seek help when they desperately need it. However, this can pose a dilemma for a nurse. Omitting relevant data from a patient's records may later be detrimental to future patient care, for example issues relating to sexual health or drug abuse.

There are, however, instances when acting in the interest of the patient may conflict with the interest of society; for example, when the information concerns the welfare of a third person who may be at risk, such as a child in a family where there is violence against another person. Clause 5.4 applies where there is an issue of child protection.

The General Medical Council requires that the practitioner should discuss the matter fully with other practitioners and if appropriate consult with a professional organisation without identifying the person concerned (Korga-onkar & Tribe 1994). If a decision is made not to disclose or provide the information in the record, it must be recorded elsewhere along with the reasons for such action and kept for future reference (UKCC 1987). However, when the patient is alcoholic, or has diabetic retinopathy, and continues to drive, the nurse has a responsibility to report this to the employer, who may then report this to the DVLC.

The question of which members of the primary healthcare team need to have access to information about a specific patient is included in Clause 5.1. It is accepted that it is impractical to gain consent every time information is shared within the team. Patients and carers must be made aware of the need for information to be shared, on occasion, with other health professionals and who those people are likely to be. In a large team there is a greater need for awareness of these issues.

The UKCC document, *Confidentiality* (1987), warned of the danger of careless talk. Sadly this basic human failing is not mentioned in later documents. Discussion of a patient's problems with a colleague in a public place, such as in an office which is open to a waiting area, or on a phone in reception, can cause confidential information to be released into the public domain and bring about complete loss of faith in the service. Even in areas that are reserved for staff, confidential details can be passed around over coffee so that information that a patient shared in confidence with one professional becomes public property.

Although many practices are paper-less, and rarely refer to the old record cards, it is essential to maintain confidentiality of data on the computer screen. This applies equally when partners attend together but do not wish their medical history to be shared, or young people attend with parents but wish to keep a previous consultation confidential.

Activity 1.1

Consider how your workplace, reception, treatment rooms, computer screens and telephones used by staff threaten confidentiality of patient information. What changes could be made to protect confidentiality?

Advertising and sponsorship

The Code warns against endorsing commercial products (Clause 7.3). A nurse may wish to recommend a blood glucose meter that she believes to be reliable in monitoring diabetes or give out health promotion leaflets or information sponsored by a drug company. This could be considered manipulation by a commercial concern or may give the impression that the profession as a body recommends a product, when other nurses might disagree (Chadwick & Tadd 1992).

It would be wise to discuss several makes of glucose meter, pointing out their advantages, disadvantages and any independent evaluation, then allow the patient to make their own choice. However, this presents problems when only specified glucose monitoring strips are prescribed from a practice formulary.

Nurses deal with people who are vulnerable and open to suggestion. It is incumbent on nurses to see that literature offered has first been read, to ensure that the message is balanced and unbiased and does not directly promote a product or a company. Also ensure the data is still relevant; old information leaflets may be incorrect. For example, leaflets discussing the benefits of hormone replacement therapy may not have been updated in line with current evidence and practice. It has to be recognised that many practices rely on support from pharmaceutical companies for health promotion literature.

Drug company sponsorship for study days and research projects is especially common to general practice. It is reasonable to assume that the valuable support of a company can lead to the advocacy of a particular product because of greater familiarity.

Activity 1.2

Consider the areas of patient care where you influence the choice of treatment. Do the drug companies who make the products you choose most frequently also provide sponsored educational events for nurses? Can you give examples of judgement swayed by commercial propaganda?

Issues of consent

The legal system in the United Kingdom requires consent from any patient who is about to undergo any treatment or surgical intervention. Without consent from the patient, the nurse or doctor delivering the care may be in danger of being sued for assault and battery. The following text relates to adults, minors and persons with a learning disability.

What is consent?

Consent to any medical or surgical intervention is a legal arrangement based on the notion of a contract between two equal parties (Alderson 1995). There is some debate as to whether equality exists between these two parties. The health professional would appear to have the upper hand by having greater knowledge of the procedure being undertaken. This may create barriers between the health professional and patient in such a way that: the patient feels coerced into something against his will; and some doctors claim it is unfair to burden patients with technicalities they would not understand.

Some patients prefer to be kept in the dark and accept a suggested treatment; others will require information about all the choices on offer, and then make a decision; while a third group will want all the information and then trust the health professional to make the right decision for them (Reeves & Orford 2002).

Although some patients may wish to take the submissive role and allow decisions to be made for them, this decision making is not the role of the health professional. Information regarding the procedure must be imparted to the patient who is then enabled to make their own decision – informed consent. This issue will be discussed later.

Express and implied consent

Consent can be given in three ways; expressly, implied or hypothetically (Reeves & Orford 2002). Express consent is usually in the form of writing, an example of which is the pre-operative consent form, but includes a nod of the head, or a verbal yes. Parents or guardians who attend with a child for vaccination would normally expect to sign a consent form.

Nurses working within general practice will usually encounter implied consent. It would be assumed that a patient who voluntarily attends a flu clinic and proffers an arm for vaccination has given implied consent to the procedure. However, women may be sent to the nurse by the doctor for vaginal swabs, but do not understand the implication of a positive chlamydia result. Hypothetical consent will rarely be encountered by the nurse, but includes an advance directive, or living will, which is discussed later in the text.

Although, legally, verbal consent is as valid as written consent, written consent is easier to produce in cases of litigation (Leung 2002), and can be scanned into patient computerised notes.

Many general practices offer training facilities, so a patient may find a student nurse, family planning student, medical student or GP registrar present during the consultation. Written consent should be obtained prior to the consultation, to give patients the opportunity to decline the observer if they so wish before they are confronted with the learner. This is particularly relevant for intimate consultations such as cervical cytology, when the woman may prefer not to have either a male or female learner in attendance.

Even if there is no objection it is important that the patient is allowed to control the flow of information. The requirements of the student must not take precedence over the need to seek consent.

Consent in English law

It is a basic rule of English law that no one has any right to touch another person without their consent. A nurse may not, therefore, do anything to a patient without obtaining their agreement. The importance of this law is to ensure that patients understand and agree to the treatment suggested. Consent must not be coerced and the benefit of any intervention must outweigh any harmful effects (Bird & White 1995).

Exceptions to this law involve some aspects of nursing care. This exception also permits the nurse to care for unconscious patients, which may be a simple faint or the need for cardio-pulmonary resuscitation in primary care.

Competence to consent

A person must be of adult years and sound mind to be capable of giving consent (Rodgers 2000). Informed consent for medical or surgical procedures may be hindered by illness, stress, mental illness or a learning disability (Chadwick & Tadd 1992). A person who is mentally incapable of understanding the nature of the treatment cannot consent to treatment. Mental competence must be assessed before obtaining valid consent. The Mental Health Act Code of Practice 1983 para. 15.10 stated that certain criteria are necessary for a person to be able to consent to treatment (Box 1.2).

If a patient is unable to give consent due to a psychological disorder, illness or stress, the relatives usually have to shoulder the burden, although the final decision will lie with the doctor. A diagnosis of mental illness does not

---

Box 1.2   The criteria necessary for a person to be able to consent (Mental Health Act 1993 para 15.10)

The patient:

1. understands what the treatment is and why he/she needs it
2. understands in broad terms the nature of the treatment
3. understands the benefits and risks
4. understands the consequences of not having the treatment
5. possesses the mental capacity to make a choice.

necessarily mean that the ability to give valid consent is affected. Fullbrook (1994) argued that the question of a patient's competence to consent to treatment is rarely raised unless there is an issue of non-compliance. He also states that the capacity to make a decision is judged in relation to the importance of the intervention. This scenario can be related to general practice. A patient who, after consultation with his general practitioner, decides against a minor surgical procedure, would have his decision respected. If this same person refuses major surgery, his mental competence could be questioned. The reader may have cared for women with advanced breast cancer who choose not to have surgery, and found it difficult to accept this decision.

Competence to consent can therefore be linked to a question of conforming. An individual has a right to make their decisions, but mental competence may be questioned if the final decision fails to conform to society's expectations. Standards may be the norm for either an individual or society. Usually when such a conflict arises the final decision is made by the person with the most authority and knowledge.

Consent for patients with learning difficulties

Mentally compromised patients are said to be unable to, or not allowed to, exercise their autonomy to its fullest extent because the ability to make autonomous decisions must be competency based (Fullbrook 1994). However, mental competence is not easily measured and may require expert analysis. This is a complex process, and in clinical practice the assessment of mental competence tends to be value judgements based on social and personal values (Hepworth 1989).

Consent for patients with severe learning difficulties, or the senile, who are regarded as incompetent to give valid consent, is usually sought from a third party. Relatives, carers or friends may be able to give an indication of the patient's wishes (Reeves & Orford 2002). Although relatives are often asked to make surrogate decisions on behalf of the patients, Fullbrook (1994) suggests that they may be mentally incompetent themselves, due to stress that may affect rational judgement.

Hanford (1993) raises ethical issues surrounding disability. She states that 'disability is rarely, if ever, given consideration in ethics teaching, even though autonomy is central to the concerns of the disabled'. This can relate to physical or mental disability. Hanford raises concerns about the moral stance professionals assume in ethical deliberations, which is central to any discussion on ethics and disability.

Nurses who care for patients with a learning disability may well have encountered the challenge of competence and consent. The three main areas of concern include immunisation, contraception and cervical cytology. These are invasive procedures that may be difficult to explain in a language the patient understands. Many of the patients who live in the community will have a key worker who has a deeper understanding of their patient's mental ability. It may be necessary to defer a procedure until the key worker can obtain the necessary consent.

A person is more likely to give valid consent if the explanation is appropriate to the level of their assessed ability (Rumbold 1993). Nurses can utilise the expertise of their learning disability nurse colleagues to ensure that patients with limited mental competence receive quality care. These nurses have the skills and tools to help the patient understand a procedure. Clause 3.6 in the Code states that criteria for treatment must be in the patient's best interests when they are not legally competent.

Informed consent

The concept of informed consent has existed for many years within the medical profession. Cadoza in 1914 stated that 'Every human being of adult years and sound mind has a right to determine what shall be done with his body; and a surgeon who performs an operation without his patient's consent commits an assault for which he is liable for damages' (cited in Rumbold 1993).

Informed consent has been defined as the patient's right to know what is entailed, before any procedure is carried out (Chadwick & Tadd 1992). This includes an explanation of any hazards or complications, and the expected final outcome of treatment. Beauchamp and Childress (2001) discuss the complexities of different commentaries about informed consent.

Simply, within general practice, it is the nurse's responsibility to ensure that the patient is fully informed about any procedure or treatment, even when they have given implied consent by attending the surgery. The patient will be competent to understand and decide voluntarily, having been given accurate information that they can understand and authorize the agreed plan of care.

The patient must be given all the relevant information in order for consent to be obtained. In England there is no actual law that stipulates how much information is given, but it is the health professional's duty to ensure that there is no undue pressure or influence on the patient. These issues emphasise the link between consent and autonomy in allowing individuals to be autonomous, and permitted to make their own decisions regarding their healthcare.

Beauchamp and Childress (2001) argue that informed consent does not exist genuinely between professional and patient, as the patient can never fully understand the information they are given. This reinforces the issue of an unequal contract between health professional and patient. As mentioned above, stress and illness may influence the patient's ability to make a rational decision even if all the information has been provided. It may be appropriate in some instances to defer a treatment until informed consent can be obtained.

Main principles of informed consent

Although some patients are unable to form an informed opinion, it must be remembered that everyone has the same rights and the two main principles must be (Rumbold 1993):

Give people the respect due to any human being
Ensure that the person is protected from harm

If a person is unable to give informed consent, it is considered good practice to discuss any proposed treatment with the next of kin (National Health Service Management Executive (NHSME) 1990), although the doctor does not have to obtain their consent as the final decision in law rests with the doctor. Failure to obtain consent or adhere to a competent refusal may result in legal action, or disciplinary proceedings against the practitioner (Rodgers 2000).

Cultural issues

Regard must be given to the cultural backgrounds within the practice population when considering informed consent in both adults and children. Difficulties with language can clearly have an impact when obtaining consent for treatment (Box 1.3). An interpreter may be required for patients whose first language is not English. This may be a child or relative, which creates problems with sensitive issues and patient confidentiality, although without an interpreter, the patient is unable to give informed consent. Access to telephone or personal interpreters is difficult and expensive, and may not be commonly considered in primary care.

Box 1.3   Examples where language barriers may prevent the nurse obtaining informed consent

- Parents who do not speak or understand English are unable to give informed consent to a procedure for their child
- Administering of vaccines, including influenza
- Prescribing diabetic medication and insulin
- Undertaking any bodily examination, including cervical smears
- Travel advice, including choice of malaria prophylaxis.

Consulting with patients with a speech or hearing disability presents similar problems, although writing information or using information leaflets can overcome some of these difficulties.

Minors and consent

A minor is legally defined as someone younger than 18 years and this is an important patient group to consider when examining issues of consent. Children are dependent on their parents or carers for their health and safety. Most parents look to health professionals to help them make the right choices to ensure that their children grow up with healthy lives. It is customary in the United Kingdom to obtain the consent of a parent or guardian before carrying out treatment on a minor, although there is no statute law stating that a child cannot give consent to, or refuse, treatment. *The Best Interest Standard* refers to the legal assumption that parents act in their children's best interests (Beauchamp & Childress 2001, p 102). To be able to consent, a parent must have sufficient information to weigh up the risks and benefits of a procedure. Failure to provide this information may lead to the consent being invalid.

It is not uncommon for a minor to refuse treatment, for example an immunisation, but the parent gives consent. Legally, if the parents have given consent the nurse may give the injection, although forcing the child to be immunised against their will could be construed criminal assault (Kline 1995). If the child fully understands the implications of the vaccine and has a valid reason for refusing, the nurse should heed the child's request.

Conversely, a child may give consent for a vaccine but the parent refuses. If the child is under 16 years, has the maturity to understand the implications and wishes to have the vaccine, the nurse may legally give the injection (Kline 1995).

The Children Act 1989, section 3(5) provides guidance for nurses dealing with emergencies in primary care when a minor is accompanied by someone without parental responsibility, for example a school teacher, or a carer. Safeguarding or promoting the child's welfare is paramount.

Activity 1.3

An unaccompanied 14-year-old boy presents in the surgery with a tetanus-prone laceration following a football injury. He is due his school leaving vaccination. Practice policy is to vaccinate only with consent of the parent or guardian. Consider the legal implications and prepare a protocol for future management of this scenario to discuss at the next practice meeting.

A competent child aged over 16 years can consent to treatment, and this cannot be overridden due to the Family Reform Act 1969 (Rodgers 2000). The subject of consent in minors was raised during the Gillick case of 1981 (Cox 1994). The issue of prescribing oral contraception to underage girls without parental consent is a major issue. Parents have duties to their children, but children also have rights. The court ruled that any parental rights were terminated when the child achieved sufficient understanding and intelligence to make an informed decision about medical treatment. This is now referred to as the *Fraser guidelines*. Children under 16 years can give valid consent to treatment if they have sufficient maturity and intelligence to understand the nature and implications of the proposed treatment (Leung 2002).

The key issue in child consent is that a child who is capable of making a reasoned decision has a right to be involved in the decision-making process. Children need to be fully informed in the same way as any other patient.

The nurse's role

Nurses can play a crucial part in helping patients to enjoy more equality with doctors in issues of consent (Box 1.4). The nurse has the ability to explain clinical information clearly and listen to patients' anxieties and concerns. Nurses also have the ability to realise that consent is an emotional and rational process (Alderson 1995). Clause 3 of the Code offers guidelines on consent. It does not dictate actions. The Code states that nurses must safeguard the interests of individual patients; the interests of the public and the patient must predominate over those of the practitioner and profession.

Legal standards of consent are based on the concept of what the reasonable doctor decides to tell the patient. A nurse who gives a patient more

---

Box 1.4   The role of the nurse in issues of consent for nursing care

The nurse should:

- use language which the patient can understand
- ensure the patient understands the procedure/treatment
- utilise an interpreter where necessary – defer a procedure unless the event is life-threatening (e.g. cardiac arrest)
- remember that children are capable of giving informed consent
- not undertake any procedure for which consent is not informed
- liase with key worker or general practitioner when mental illness or incapacity prevents the patient giving informed consent

information about the risks than the doctor wishes could be placed in a difficult position (Rumbold 1993), but withholding information is contrary to the NMC guidelines.

Respect for patient autonomy in general practice

It is essential that healthcare workers understand the concept of autonomy, in order to individualise healthcare. Although the terms autonomy and self-determination are often used interchangeably in ethical textbooks, autonomy will be used throughout the following text. This section will consider the general issues of autonomy pertinent to practice nurses.

What is autonomy?

Autonomy is derived from the Greek *autos* (self) and *nomos* (rule, governance or law) (Beauchamp & Childress 2001, p 57). An autonomous person has the ability to be able to choose for themselves or more extensively to be able to formulate and carry out their own plans or policies. The autonomous person also has the ability to govern their conduct by rules and values, and is said to be self-determining.

Activity 1.4

Reflect on a recent situation in your practice when a patient was not involved in their treatment plan. An example of this could be in respiratory care, when the choice of inhaler device is reliant on the practice drug formulary. Do they have a choice of inhaler device? Consider how this situation could have been managed to enable the individual to exert their autonomy.

Ethical issues

The principle of autonomy is commonly regarded as the first principle of contemporary biomedical ethics. Within healthcare autonomy can only occur if the patient has at their disposal the necessary information to consider a course of treatment consistent with their beliefs and wishes. Nurses are also autonomous people who do not blindly follow orders but respect their patients' wishes. Autonomy of the nurse and autonomy of the patient appear to be increasingly interdependent.

The principles of autonomy and individuality would suggest that patients should be entitled to information about their condition. Bird and White (1995) suggest that healthcare professionals must provide all the appropriate information required by a prudent patient to make an informed choice, even when it is not requested. This is contrary to the belief that it is a denial of autonomy to force unwanted information on those who have clearly indicated that they do not want it (Lindley 1991). The patient is now required to read and sign a consent form, which mentions risks of the procedure, prior to minor surgery. If the patient fails to read the form he is qualified to act autonomously, but fails to do so (Beauchamp and Childress 2001).

Sharing information with patients

Healthcare professionals have a moral obligation to give patients as much unbiased information as possible with which to make informed autonomous decisions (Rowson 1993). Seedhouse (1998) discusses autonomy as a quality, making the distinction between *creating autonomy* and *respecting autonomy*. It is not possible for someone to make a decision of their own free will if they do not know the options open to them.

It is unfortunate that some professionals consider it morally acceptable to give selected information to a patient, believing it to be in the best interests of the patient to do so. This may deny the individual a chance to make an informed choice, reduce his autonomy and increase anxiety. An example of this is when discussing a new medication. If the prescriber fails to explain the potential risks/benefits of medication options, patient autonomy is reduced. This may result in a loss of trust and confidence in the profession. It is hoped that nurse prescribers will redress this with their prescribing practice.

Refusal to disclose relevant information may deprive people of the power to make important decisions affecting their lives. This leads to dilemma in truth telling. Where a doctor fails to answer questions about diagnosis and prognosis truthfully, the nurse is expected to refer these questions back to the practitioner. She may, however, feel comfortable to field some questions by determining the patient's current knowledge and then answer appropriately. Relevant internet websites, help lines or societies such as the Parkinson's Society, may be useful resources for patients to gain more in-depth knowledge about their condition, treatment options and prognosis.

Although there may be occasions when beneficence overrides respect for autonomy, such as. acting for the patient's good, there should be few occasions for this to affect nursing care. These issues may become more relevant as the nurse's role in general practice expands.

Activity 1.5

Mr White is a 55-year-old manual worker. During a routine health check you discover that his blood pressure is 170/110 mm/Hg. He asks you what this means and if this is serious. Consider what information you want Mr White to share with you, and what you are competent and comfortable to share with him. You may achieve increased compliance in lifestyle management if you discuss the implications of unmanaged hypertension. You may, however, increase his anxiety. Justify your decision to share or withhold unbiased information from your patient.

Consent and autonomy

Informed consent and autonomy are linked by the presumption that mature adults are expected to be mentally competent and have a capacity for autonomy. There is a moral requirement to show respect for this autonomy.

If the patient has the capacity it is necessary to ensure that they understand the nature and consequences of a choice. Efforts to dissuade the patient are acceptable, and even morally obligatory in some instances. The nurse has a role to help family and carers to come to terms with a patient's choice and to respect it.

A concern with patient autonomy as an ethical issue can pose problems in the delivery of care. Wright and Levac (1992) consider that it is arrogant, insulting and violent to label families as noncompliant when they do not respond to nursing intervention.

Activity 1.6

The practice receives points for administering influenza vaccine to patients in at risk groups every year. The flu campaign targets these patients with an invitation, then a phone call. The patient is reminded at every consultation. The patient notes are flagged. Consider the ethical implications of this policy. Devise an argument to present to the practice meeting for respecting patients' autonomy. This may require a modification in the initial policy.

Suggestion: eligible patients have an information leaflet and/or discussion about the vaccine benefits and side effects. The patient can then make an informed decision whether or not to accept the offer. This decision should be respected.

It is important that the individual is able to make a voluntary decision about their treatment. Consent obtained through coercion or manipulation is not regarded as true consent. Manipulation includes giving information to influence the individual, or withholding information that alters a person's understanding. This is then not informed consent. It could be argued that, in some instances, nurses who encourage parents to allow their children to be vaccinated have used an element of (unintentional) manipulation to achieve this result.

The nonautonomous patient

Some people prefer not to make a decision about their treatment and rely on the doctor or nurse to make that decision. These people are described as being nonautonomous. Seedhouse (1998) suggests that many people are content to be instructed although independent choosing should be encouraged. If it is clear that it is the patient's own wish to leave the decision making to the professional, this decision should be respected. A patient who is very ill may choose to be nonautonomous only until their health improves.

Refusal of treatment

An action of battery is a legal suit that may be brought against a nurse if treatment is given in the face of an explicit refusal to treatment (McHale 1995). There is no power in statute or case law to remove a patient to hospital for treatment unless they fall under the Mental Health Act 1983. Where a patient declines care, the refusal should be respected. Although it is hoped that practice nurses would not encounter this scenario they must be aware of the implications of such action. Examples of refusal of treatment include choosing not to take medication for hypertension, even when there is a risk of a stroke, and not taking preventative asthma medication despite needing regular reliever therapy.

Patient autonomy and the practice nurse

It would appear that patients and their families are now more informed regarding healthcare and patient rights. The *Patients' Charter* (DH 1993) developed an increased awareness of a person's right to self-determination. Health related topics regularly appear in national and local newspapers and in many weekly and monthly magazines. Media articles and access to the internet have resulted in many more people questioning proposed and current treatment options, and they attend the surgery armed with internet print-outs and media articles. There is an increasing expectation that decision making should be both fully informed and collaborative. Healthcare professionals have come to recognise and respect the autonomy of individuals, moving away from prescriptive management towards a negotiated contract of care.

Essentially all nursing actions invade a person's privacy, and although most of these actions are considered necessary, and consent is given implicitly, it should not be taken for granted. The patient should be allowed to exercise the right to say no.

Involving patients in making decisions is said to improve health and promote patient welfare (Chadwick & Tadd 1992). Real care involves a partnership of nurse and patient/patient. Chadwick and Tadd suggest that using the word client instead of patient implies that the person receiving care is an autonomous chooser. It could be argued that a client is a person who is paying for a service. Within healthcare, private patients pay at the point of use, while those receiving National Health Service treatment pay through their national insurance contributions.

Patients from higher social classes receive more explanations voluntarily than those from lower social classes, although demand for information and advice is widespread among all social groups (Townsend, Davidson & Whitehead 1992). This issue may need addressing to ensure that all patients are empowered to be autonomous, whatever their social group, ethnicity or disability.

Patients should be offered information, which if accepted, must be delivered at a level the patient and family/carer can understand, with audio-visual or written support for patients to read and absorb at their own pace.

Refusal to consent is an area that may cause concern within general practice. Patients who refuse to attend reviews for certain conditions can now be exempted from target figures. Harassing patients in order to achieve targets violates their autonomy and should be discouraged. Although the advantages of encouraging patient autonomy are recognised, there are several reasons why nurses may be reluctant to encourage such participation (Box 1.5) (Saunders 1995).

Encouraging autonomy is time consuming, but can result in improved treatment concordance that may save further surgery appointments and/or reduce patient morbidity (Edwards 1996).

Conversely, it could be argued that patients are denied autonomy when they cannot access a drug or treatment, due to financial restraints in the practice or health service budget. In the case of new drugs which are promoted in the media, an open discussion about risk/benefits of these products

---

Box 1.5   Reasons why nurses may be reluctant to encourage patient autonomy

These include:

- feeling threatened by the patient having a stronger role in the partnership
- being asked too many questions
- patients should put their trust in the nursing and medical staff
- fear that the nurse's role will be eroded as more patients self-care
- tasks are completed faster and more thoroughly if the patient remains a passive recipient of care.

---

can reassure the patient, who may be happy to continue with their current prescribed treatment.

Autonomy in health promotion

Although lay people need to develop the confidence and competence to take responsibility for their own health, the whole concept of health education raises ethical questions. Banning smoking in public places has created a regular debate in the media and nursing press. The proposed policies take no account of patient choice.

Health educators have to respect the rights and autonomy of the individual to choose their lifestyle, despite the primary remit for the prevention of disease (see Chapter 4). Health promotion features strongly in a general practice workload. Advice on lifestyle changes must be individualised and sensitive, respecting the patient's culture and social values. The role of the nurse includes spending time with the patient identifying their social norms and values. A person who makes an informed decision not to follow a healthy lifestyle following a health screening programme should have their decision respected, even when this may impact negatively on their future health. Nurses can only inform and advise.

Advocacy and autonomy

Gates (1994) addressed many of the arguments surrounding advocacy and nursing. As an advocate for autonomy, the nurse assists the patient to make an authentic decision that meets their own values and lifestyle. The nurse may also act as the patient's advocate if decisions made by others conflict with the person's wishes. If a nurse is unable to act on a patient's behalf, the patient should be referred to a local independent advocacy scheme. Each Primary Care Trust has a Patient Advocacy Liaison Service (PALS), to which the patient can be referred, and who will act for the patient.

Autonomy and trainees

Thompson, Melia and Boyd (1994) discussed the ethical issues of using patients during nurse or doctor training. Students, doctors and nurses receive training in general practice. They develop many skills, including taking cervical smears and minor surgery. Patients may be uncomfortable with the thought they are 'on camera' during videoed consultations during registrar training due to lack of understanding. It should be explained to the patient that it is the doctor who is being recorded, and not the patient.

Patients should be allowed to consent or refuse examination or treatment by a learner even when this restricts training opportunities, without this decision affecting future care and with permission sought prior to the learner meeting the patient.

Living wills (advance directives)

Living wills are recognised as valid documents in civil law. They are advance directives that allow patients to take some control over end-of-life decisions. This includes refusal of treatment in advance or to state their preference for treatment to continue should they become too ill to make their own choice or to express that choice. Practice nurses are unlikely to follow advance directives within their professional role, but may be asked to read, witness or discuss the concept of the living will during a consultation.

A major advantage of living wills is that they can promote discussion, especially when broaching difficult subjects (Haas 2005). Practice nurses often have a close rapport with their patients, and may be the person the patient approaches to discuss sensitive issues.

The Mental Capacity Act (2007) allows patients to choose their end-of-life care. These decisions may be discussed in practice meetings, or cancer care team meetings, so it is helpful for the nurse to be forewarned. An advance statement only comes into force when a patient is unable to make decisions.

Summary

Effective decision making is an integral part of the clinical role of the practitioner, involving risk taking within the parameters of the professional accountability placed on each registered nurse. Indeed, the *Report of the Heathrow Debate* (Department of Health 1994, p308) reiterates a comment that 'nurses will not have arrived until they are sued'. It is hoped that this will not be the case.

The professional trend towards negotiated, autonomous nurse–patient healthcare has enabled a move away from the old paternalistic methods, where health professionals knew what was best for the patient, although it is important to recognise that some patients still prefer to follow instructions without information, accepting the doctor's or nurse's advice. The patient's role is changing from one of grateful recipient to active consumer. It has been argued that although completely autonomous decision making is a myth, the person seeking the informed consent should allow the individual the freedom to make their own choice, although deciding a person's autonomous interests is a difficult matter.

Clause 3.2 of the Code reinforces the nurses' role in respecting patients' involvement in planning and delivery of care. Nurses have a duty to inform patients of their rights and assist them to ask questions and express their opinions. Nurses who are not comfortable in this role may benefit from reflection and training to develop the necessary skills to fulfil this duty.

The nurse has a duty to respect patients who prefer to be nonautonomous and passive in their care, preferring the nurse or doctor to make all the decisions about their care. Patients should be offered information about their disease, treatment and general management, and allowed to accept or reject this offer (Figure 1.3).

One of the central aims of nursing in 2008 and beyond is the development of autonomous practitioners who are better able to assist patients to cope and take decisions. Individualised patient care recognises the patient as a person, and not as an object of clinical practice. The fear of patient litigation may increase patient autonomy in the future. Respect for the individual requires that each person must be treated as unique and as an equal to every other person. There are few areas where a person cannot, if they choose, be autonomous in their healthcare.

Key points

- The Code lays a moral responsibility rather than a statutory duty on members of the profession
- The Code makes the practitioner responsible for maintaining and developing their knowledge, skill and competence
- A person must be fully informed to be able to consent to a procedure or treatment

- A person must have the mental capacity in order to be fully informed
- Children have a right to be involved in their healthcare
- Treatment without consent may be considered assault
- Some patients prefer to be nonautonomous
- The nurse must respect a decision to refuse care or treatment
- The nurse may need to act as advocate to enable a patient to assert their autonomy.

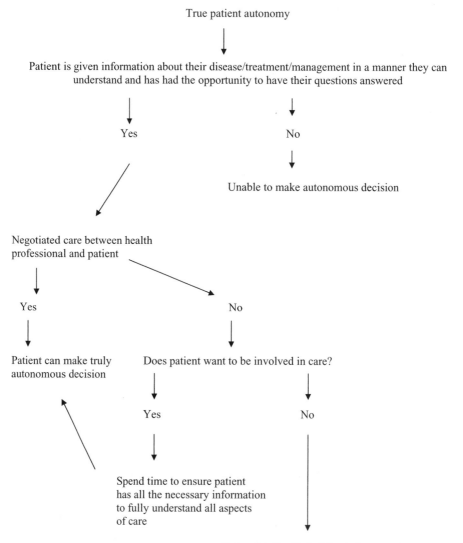

Figure 1.3   True patient autonomy.

Recommended reading

Beauchamp T & Childress J (2001) *Principles of Biomedical Ethics 5th Edn.* New York: Oxford University Press.

Jones M (1996) *Accountability in Practice: A Guide to Professional Responsibility for Nurses in Practice.* Salisbury: Quay Books.

Seedhouse D (1998) *Ethics the Heart of Health Care 2nd Edn.* Chichester: John Wiley & Sons.

References

Alderson P (1995) Consent to surgery: the role of the nurse *Nursing Standard* 9(8), 38–40.

Beauchamp T & Childress J (2001) *Principles of Biomedical Ethics 5th edn.* New York: Oxford University Press.

Bergman R (1981) Accountability: Definition and Dimensions. *International Nursing Review* 28(2), 53–59.

Bird A & White J (1995) Consent and the adult patient. An ethical perspective – patient autonomy. In Tingle J & Cribb A (Eds). *Nursing Law and Ethics.* Oxford: Blackwell Science.

Burnard P & Chapman C M (1988) *Professional and Ethical Issues in Nursing.* Chichester: John Wiley & Sons.

Castledine G (1992) New Code of Professional Conduct: how it affects you. *British Journal of Nursing* 1(6), 296–300

Chadwick R & Tadd W (1992) *Ethics and Nursing Practice* London: Macmillan.

Cox D (1994) Ethics and the law *G.P.* Sept, 44–46.

Department of Health (1993) *The Patients' Charter.* London: HMSO.

Department of Health (1994) *The Heathrow Debate 1993: The Challenges for Nursing and Midwifery in the 21st Century.* London: HMSO.

Edwards M (1996) Drug Compliance: a continuing problem. *Practice Nursing.* 7(20), 21–22.

Evans A (1993) Accountability: a core concept for primary nursing. *Journal of Clinical Nursing* 2, 231–234.

Fullbrook P (1994) Assessing mental competence of patients and relatives. *Journal of Advanced Nursing* 20, 457–461.

Gates B (1994) *Advocacy. A Nurses Guide.* London: Scutari Press.

Hanford L (1993) Ethics and disability. *British Journal of Nursing.* 2(19), 979–982.

Haas F (2005) Understanding the legal implications of living wills. *Nursing Times* 101(3), 34–37.

Hepworth S (1989) Professional judgement and nurse education. *Nurse Education Today* 9, 408–412.

Holland S (2004) *Introducing Nursing Ethics. Themes in Theory and Practice.* Salisbury: APS Publishing.

Jones M (1996) *Accountability in Practice: A Guide to Professional Responsibility for Nurses in General Practice.* Salisbury: Quay Books.

Kline R (1995) Immunisation: at the sharp end. *Health Visitor* 68(10), 412.

Korgaonkar G & Tribe D (1994) Confidentiality, patients and the law. *British Journal of Nursing* 3(2), 91–93.

Leung WC (2002) Consent to treatment in the A & E department. *Accident and Emergency Nursing* 10, 17–25.

Lindley R (1991) Informed consent and the ghost of Bolam. In: Brazier M and Lobjoit M (Eds). *Protecting the Vulnerable. Autonomy and Consent in Health Care.* London: Routledge.

McHale J (1995) Consent and the adult patient. The legal perspective. In Tingle J and Cribb A (Eds). *Nursing Law and Ethics. Oxford*: Blackwell Science.

National Health Service Management Executive (1990) *A Guide to Consent for Examination or Treatment.* London: NHMSE.

Nursing and Midwifery Council (2004) *The Code of Professional Conduct: Standards for Conduct, Performance and Ethics.* London: NMC.

Nursing and Midwifery Council (2007) New Code – coming soon! *NMC News*, 4.

Pyne R (1992) Accountability in principle and in practice. *British Journal of Nursing* 1(6), 304.

Pyne R (1994) Empowerment through use of the Code of Professional Conduct. *British Journal of Nursing* 3(12), 631–634.

Reeves M & Orford J (2002) *Fundamental Aspects of Legal, Ethical and Professional Issues in Nursing.* London: Quay Books.

Rodgers ME (2000) The child patient and consent to treatment: legal overview. *British Journal of Community Nursing* 5(10), 494–498.

Rowson R (1993) Informed consent. In Tschudin V (Ed.). *Ethics, Nurses and Patients.* London: Scutari Press.

Rumbold G (1993) *Ethics in Nursing Practice.* London: Bailliere Tindall.

Saunders P (1995) Encouraging patients to take part in their own care. *Nursing Times* 91(5), 42–43.

Seedhouse D (1998) *Ethics: The Heart of Healthcare 2nd edn.* Chichester: John Wiley & Sons.

Tadd V (1994) Professional codes: an exercise in tokenism? *Nursing Ethics* 1(1), 15–23.

Thiroux J (1980) *Ethics, Theory and Practice 2nd Edn.* Encino, CA: Glencoe Publishing.

Thompson IA, Melia KM & Boyd KM (1994) *Nursing Ethics 3rd Edn.* London: Churchill Livingstone.

Townsend P, Davidson N & Whitehead M (1992) *Inequalities in Health.* London: Penguin.

Tschudin V (1994a) Nursing Ethics 4: Theories and Principles. *Nursing Standard* 9(2), 52–55.

Tschudin V (1994b) Nursing Ethics 6: Particular Features. *Nursing Standard* 9(4), 52–55.

United Kingdom Central Council for Nursing, Midwifery and Health Visiting (1987) *Confidentiality: A UKCC Advisory Paper.* London: UKCC.

United Kingdom Central Council for Nursing, Midwifery and Health Visiting (1989) *Exercising Accountability: A UKCC Advisory Document.* London: UKCC.

United Kingdom Central Council for Nursing, Midwifery and Health Visiting (1992) *The Scope of Professional Practice.* London: UKCC.

Wright LM and Levac AMC (1992) The non-existence of non-compliant families: the influence of Humberto Maturana. *Journal of Advanced Nursing* 17(8), 913–917.

Young AP (1989) *Legal Problems in Nursing Practice.* London: Chapman & Hall.

Chapter 2

Management

Pat Tweed, Marilyn Edwards and Karen Mayne

An understanding of the culture and structure of organisations offers an insight into some of the difficulties the reader may encounter within the workplace. Although this may appear to be a complex subject, each aspect is broken down into comprehensible sections to which the reader can relate. It is hoped that this chapter may encourage each nurse to look objectively at their employing organisation and be involved in a team/practice management plan.

Change is inevitable, and is inherent in the modern National Health Service. It is integral to all aspects of the nurse's work. An example of this is offered, to encourage readers to become more involved in their organisation. The effective management of an organisation includes time management and clinical governance issues. This chapter examines time management in general practice, and, though the emphasis is on the role of the practice nurse, it has repercussions for all the staff. Clinical governance relates to quality in meeting the needs of all the people in the system. This includes appreciation of risk management and audit. The latter can provide the evidence of efficient and effective quality healthcare practice that meets the goals and objectives of the organisation. Management issues relate to all aspects of nursing actions and are incorporated into subsequent chapters where relevant.

Organisations

All organisations have a structure, even if none is apparent. Drucker (1974) states that structure is a means for obtaining the objectives and goals of an organisation. This section will look at different cultures that exist in organisations and the way in which these are reflected in the management structures of general practice, where internal and external factors have combined to influence that structure in recent years.

The Informed Practice Nurse, Edwards, M. (2008), Chichester: Wiley.

Authority, leadership and autonomy

Authority is related to status and it implies a right to control and judge the action of others, while leadership is the exercise of the power conferred by that right (Torrington & Weightman 1989). A leader may inspire through the shaping and sharing of a vision, described by Macgregor Burns (1978) as transformational leadership; or results may be achieved through allowing the follower to know what is expected and trusting them to achieve it. Autonomy is the freedom of action that subordinates see as being necessary to be effective in their roles.

Consideration of current organisational structures may enable the reader to recognise the prevailing culture of their organisation and how to work more effectively within it, seek to change it or even to recognise the incompatibility of personal beliefs and those of an employer. Handy (1993) suggested that cultures stem from deeply held beliefs about the organisation of work, the exercise of authority and how people should be rewarded and controlled. Cultures are founded and built by the dominant groups in an organisation and their appropriateness will change as the people within the groups and their relative power changes. This can be seen in many general practices where the combination of the organisational changes in the NHS, increased patient expectation and the vast expansion of screening and preventative health services have overturned the existing culture, and the former management structure has not been adequately replaced.

Technology and organisational cultures

The technology of an organisation greatly influences its structure. General practice is a combination of routine and nonroutine work, the former according to Handy (1993) being more generally suited to a role culture and the latter to a power or task culture. Routine, programmable operations such as screening and immunisation are most effectively carried out within a hierarchical structure, in which the work is controlled by policies and protocols, and the areas of discretion are narrow.

However, the individualised care needed for encouragement of lifestyle change or dealing with chronic disease, are more suited to a matrix structure based on teams that incorporate nurses, doctors and other health and social care professionals, with a variety of expertise. General practice also requires the ability to deal with rapidly changing and emergency situations, when there is no time to wait for instructions or to discuss with team colleagues. Decisions must be made and action taken independently by confident and competent individuals who are more likely to be found within a power culture, where they are used to being trusted to get on with the job (Handy

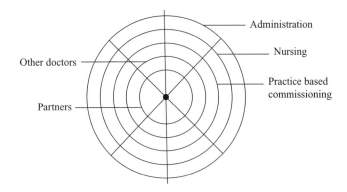

Figure 2.1 Power culture (adapted from Handy 1993).

1993). The vastly differing range of technologies and personality types in a small organisation such as general practice may be a significant deterrent to the formulation of a common management structure.

Handy (1993) identified four main types of organisational culture (Box 2.1). The power and task cultures are closely related to those described by Schein (1986) in his conceptual studies of organisations, as Organisation 'A', where ideas come from individuals and people are considered responsible, motivated and capable of governing themselves. The role culture equates with Schein's Organisation 'B', where truth comes from older, wiser and higher-status members and staff loyally carry out directions. The person culture usually has no identifiable organisational structure, but is often seen as a cluster of individuals.

Box 2.1   Organisational cultures and structures (Handy 1993)

culture	*structure*
power	web
role	Greek temple
task	matrix (net)
person	cluster

Power culture

This culture is usually found in small, entrepreneurial organisations where the structure is a web with a central power source (Figure 2.1), usually derived from the personality of the leader. This could be the senior partner in a general medical practice.

Rays of power and influence radiate from the centre connected by functional or specialist strings (nursing, administrative or financial), each co-ordinated by a key individual. Effectiveness depends on the person in the centre and the selection of power-orientated, politically minded risk-takers in the functional strings who are allowed to get on with the job.

These cultures judge by results and are tolerant of means; there are few rules or procedures and little bureaucracy. Lines of communication are often informal and run between the centre and the co-ordinators. The atmosphere is competitive and progress for the individual is through horizontal tracking (Handy 1991).

More of the same work or different work at the same level allows for development of wider expertise, as there are few opportunities for vertical promotion in such a structure. This type of structure can be found in some general practices. However, many of the people who have worked in public services such as health find this type of structure demoralising and difficult to understand, either due to its lack of formal rules, hierarchies and systems of communication, or because of a psychological attachment to the underlying culture and a lack of understanding of management.

The central person needs to choose people who think the same way as themselves, to ensure that the objectives of the organisation, or the centre's personal objectives, will be achieved with the minimum of bureaucracy or need for central control over processes. Such organisations have the ability to move quickly when threatened, which in the current climate of discontinuous change can enable them to take advantage of immediate opportunities, but this will only happen if there is strong central leadership. In a web structure the vision will not be realised without the right choice of key individuals in the specialist strings.

The role culture

The role culture, with its representative structure of a Greek temple (Figure 2.2), is dependent on the strength of its pillars; in health service organisations these might be finance, administration, medicine and nursing.

The pillars are co-ordinated at the top by a narrow band of senior management, and the work of the pillars is controlled by rules and procedures, which if followed, will ensure the result. The job description or role is often more important than the person who fulfils it (Handy 1993). This perception does little to encourage extra effort or innovation; indeed these are often actively discouraged. Influence comes from the position held and not from expertise or personality.

Communication is clear and vertical, usually top-down, with lots of paperwork. Though the system tends to be slow and unwieldy, it provides security

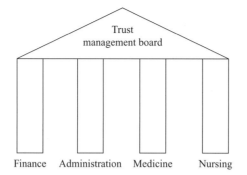

Figure 2.2 Role culture – the temple (adapted from Handy 1993).

and visible advancement up the ladder. Role culture is common in the hospital services, particularly since the introduction of hospital Trusts. It is not common in general practice largely due to the small size and absence of rules and established procedures, but this may change. Practices with many partners may follow this management style.

The growing enthusiasm for Managed Care Programmes that promote only evidence-based treatments would be most easily applied in such a structure. Doctors and nurses work to defined protocols and procedures. These are task-oriented, providing only proven cost-effective treatment, with little respect for the value of experience and professional skill.

The task culture

The task culture seeks to bring together the appropriate people and resources to do the job and, with its emphasis on results, teamwork and devolution of power, it is most in tune with current ideologies, a view supported by Handy (1993).

Influence is expert rather than personal or positional. It is also more widely distributed so that each member of the team feels more empowered. Teams, task forces and project groups are formed for a purpose and disbanded or reformed when the task is complete. The accompanying structure is a matrix or net (Figure 2.3) and the power and influence lies at the knots of the net where the relevant resources and expertise meet.

Communication is horizontal and vertical, and may be problematic if different directorates or professional groups have differing philosophies or internal structures. Authority is devolved to the grass roots, with fewer procedures and a flattened hierarchy. The increasing movement towards a primary care based NHS, which is likely to continue whatever the prevailing political mood, highlights the contribution to be made to healthcare by

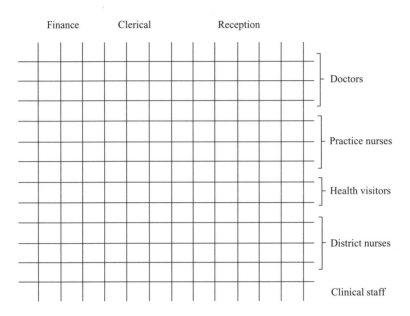

Figure 2.3 Task culture – the matrix (adapted from Handy 1993). Appropriate staff with necessary levels authority come together as a team to complete a task.

nonmedical members of the primary healthcare team. This may be through practice-based commissioning (Department of Health 2006a), which allow practices to manage all their resources to purchase healthcare. Task culture would give the necessary flexibility to develop team working and provide a more exciting and fulfilling career path for primary care nurses. This flexibility could permit a group to be formed in a practice to develop a strategy for the prevention of coronary heart disease, which may need to change its membership when it moves to set standards for the control of hyperlipidaemia, when different expertise is needed.

The person culture

The individual is the central point within the person culture. The structure, if one exists, serves only to assist the individuals within it.

Handy (1993) defines the psychological contract, as stating that 'the organisation is subordinate to the individual and depends on the individual for its existence'. If such individuals decide to band together for the furtherance of a mutual interest, the structure (the group practice), would resemble a loose cluster. This culture has existed in professional practices of architects, solicitors and more recently in general medical practice. Some single-handed doctors have formed partnerships of independent contractors providing an individualistic service to a group of patients, supported by ancillary staff, which includes nurses. This is the preferred culture of many general practitioners. The power base is expert and individuals 'do what they are good at': a situation described by Strong and Robinson (1990) as rampant individualism. Authority is generally seen as being related to superior status – in this case that of the professional, the doctor.

The change in political climate has forced change on doctors, who are now obliged to operate in a different type of organisation. This has provided nursing with the opportunity to ensure that its contribution is recognised by doctors and other primary care professionals.

Activity 2.1

Identify the culture reflected in the structure of your organisation. Which type of technology does your practice deal with best? Is it the routine programmable work, the individual teamwork or the emergency, crisis interventions? Does your assessment of the culture appear to fit?

The reader is now asked to consider the challenges of change management within a task culture, and place it in context of their own working environment.

Change management

Change management involves moving from A to B efficiently and effectively (Handy 1993). Although directives in healthcare are usually government led, the process of delivery is left to each general practice, which then develops its own method of change. The following text describes one change management process, led by a practice nurse, which can be adapted as a template for nurses wishing to develop a strategy of their own.

The change agent

A leader (change agent) is required to manage the change process; the role being to plan, prioritise, set the direction, allocate work, delegate and control (Armstrong 2001). A successful change agent will have high task orientation and person-centred leadership skills, which is consistent with action-centred leadership (Adair 1988a). Appropriate listening and communication skills are required, combined with a commitment to a vision (Broome 1990), and a commitment to develop and motivate individuals within their organisation (Workforce and Development Leadership Working Group 2000). The key elements necessary for effective leadership are listed in Box 2.2.

Box 2.2   The key elements of the functional approach to effective leadership (Adair 1988a)

defining the task	evaluating
planning	motivating
briefing	organising
controlling	setting an example

Data collection

It was noted over 30 years ago that hand washing alone was not effective in preventing patient infection (Ojajarvi, Makela & Rantasalo 1977). The National Patient Safety Agency (2004) provided guidelines for clinicians to use alcohol hand gel where the hands are not visibly soiled as best evidence-based practice. The change agent gathered evidence visually and orally and confirmed that 100% of clinicians within the practice were not using alcohol hand gel. This was due to lack of knowledge and no hand gel being available.

Diagnosis of the problem

As there was no local study on post-operative infection within general practice, the target for this change management strategy was to provide adequate training and change the process of hand washing, following overwhelming national and international evidence (Girou, Loyeau, Legrand, Oppein & Brun-Boisson 2002; Ojajarvi 2003; Strauss, Stephen, Sonnex & Gray 2003).

Solution

It would be unacceptable to maintain current hand-washing practices in the light of the evidence and government guidelines. One solution could be to wash hands more frequently, although this is unsupported by the evidence, and could potentially lead to occupationally acquired skin disorders. The only reasonable solution was to use alcohol hand gel appropriately in clinical practice. The project aims were:

1. to develop a protocol for using alcohol hand gel by all staff involved in clinical patient care
2. to evaluate the use by measuring staff satisfaction, financial costs and monitoring practice by staff and patient questionnaire

3. to promote long-term sustainability of use by developing a culture of evidence-based practice.

Implementation

A situation analysis was carried out to identify barriers, levers and facilitators to change (Kanter 1983). The change agent discussed this extensively with the specialist infection control nurse.

Lewin's force field analysis (Lewin 1951) was used to predict success of the project. Risks included financial issues and occupational health and safety. The practice partners agreed the financial risk was small. There was no evidence to support long-term exposure to hand gel posing a risk to healthcare workers. Staff acceptance and capability was considered and an open meeting of all clinicians held to introduce the procedure change. This was an opportunity for staff to question and discuss any concerns, with published evidence available for those who requested it. This process developed a model of group-decision making (King & Anderson, 2002; Sullivan & Decker 1997) and to pre-empt resistance by encouraging participation and involvement (Kotter & Schleslinger 1979). Hand hygiene was discussed with the group, recognising the ineffectiveness of one-off educational interventions (Naikoba & Hayward 2001), and the fact that the degree of knowledge does not necessarily predict appropriate behaviour (Alvaran, Butz & Larson 1994).

Following the event, supplies of hand gel were purchased and staff began to replace appropriate hand-washing events with the use of gel. Written feedback gave positive reinforcement of the change.

Resistance

A contingency approach was taken to overcome anticipated resistance (Kotter & Schleslinger, 1979), involving the senior partner from the beginning of the change process, and having regular discussions with all the practice doctors. This was a meaningful partnership theory to encourage relationship building and working with others (Murray 2000).

Evaluation

The aim of evaluation was to assess whether the change was working in practice (Tiffany & Lutjens, 1998). The change agent tested the clinician's knowledge verbally and ensured that alcohol gel was available in all clinical rooms. The financial cost of the gel was measured after six months by audit, and stocks were continually monitored as a measurement of use. Staff satisfaction was measured by questionnaire. All staff felt satisfied that they were informed regarding the change process and felt confident to probe the change agent at any time during the change over. All staff reported complete satisfaction with the use of hand gel.

Activity 2.2

Consider an area within your practice that you would like to change. Plan your change process, using yourself as the change agent. What is the project? Who else will be involved? What is the timescale? How will you evaluate it?

Clinical governance in general practice

Clinical governance refers to any strategy that ensures that local delivery of care is continuously improved to safeguard standards of care (Royal College of Nursing 2003). The RCN (2003) also states that public and patient involvement is an essential requirement for effective clinical governance. Wall, Gerada, Conlon, Ombler-Spain and Warner (2006) state that clinical governance aims to raise patients' expectations about the quality and safety of their care, to make clinicians more accountable for their actions, to increase job satisfaction for professionals, to improve clinical outcomes, and reduce significant incidents and errors.

Clinical governance means developing a structured system so that looking at the quality of care is an everyday part of life in a GP practice (Simpson 2002). The reader is directed to Van Zwanenberg and Harrison (2004) for a clear insight into clinical governance in primary care.

Duty of care

Nurses have a legal and professional duty to care for patients (Nursing and Midwifery Council 2004). Despite the increasingly limited resources at the disposal of health service workers, every practitioner has a responsibility for ensuring patients receive a high level of quality care. Lifelong learning and personal development are integral to delivering this care (Simpson 2002).

Quality assurance

The purpose of quality assurance is to ensure the consumer receives nursing of a specified degree of excellence through continuous measurement and evaluation (Schmadl, quoted in Sale 1996, p13).

Quality assurance measures the actual level of service provided and is a means of offering an efficient, cost-effective service. This includes efforts to modify provision of these services where appropriate. For example, an audit of patient waiting times may suggest a modification of the surgery appointment system. Many examples of quality assurance tools can be found in textbooks; the reader is directed to further reading (at the end of this chapter) for in-depth analysis of the topic.

Measuring quality

The six measurable areas, related to general practice, that can be addressed to ensure quality in healthcare (Ranade 1994) are described below.

1. Appropriateness: the service or procedure is one that the individual or population actually needs. A practice profile will highlight the social and ethnic mix of your population (Chapter 4).
2. Equity: services are fairly shared among the population who need them. There is documented evidence of inequality in healthcare between social groups (Townsend, Whitehead & Davidson 1992). Efforts have been made to redress some of these inequities; devising, maintaining and utilising a register for people with a learning disability can lead to improved inclusion in all aspects of healthcare.
3. Accessibility: services are readily accessible and not compromised by distance or time restraints. Surgeries that operate from 9am till 5pm are not accessible for commuters or manual workers who often work long hours.
4. Effectiveness: the services achieve the intended benefit for the individual and for the population. This can be assessed through clinical audit (see later text).
5. Acceptability: the service satisfies the reasonable expectations of patients, providers and the community. Satisfaction may be viewed subjectively, as individuals' expectations can vary according to race, social group, and education.
6. Efficiency: resources are not wasted on one service or patient to the detriment of another. Self-care, for example in wound management, is an efficient use of resources for some patients in some instances.

Activity 2.3

Choose one area of patient care, for example, prevention of coronary heart disease, and consider whether it meets the six criteria described above. This may help you identify areas for future standard setting and clinical audit.

Donabedian (1988) suggests that scientific measurement be used where possible, supplementing quantitative measures with qualitative data. His work relates to the theory of structure, process and outcome, which can be applied to many areas of healthcare (see Figure 2.4).

STRUCTURE

teamwork, resources, training

PROCESS

standards, negotiated patient care

OUTCOME

feedback - subjective or objective

clinical audit

PROFESSIONAL EXPECTATION   PATIENT EXPECTATION

how do these vary?

Figure 2.4   Simplified example of quality assurance.

- **Structure** encompasses material and human resources, and includes the environment, supplies, and all levels of staff. It can also include methods of peer review and methods of reimbursement.
- **Process** denotes what is actually done in giving and receiving care, including the patient's activities in seeking care as well as the practitioner's activities in making a diagnosis.
- **Outcome** denotes the effects of care on the patient. Outcome measures reflect total care received, are readily understood, and can be used to indicate not just quality of care, but needs for further or compensatory care. Specified outcomes provide the feedback for future care.

Attree (1993) explored the concept of quality, and offered a framework for quality care that includes Donabedian's principles. Structural criteria included organisational variables, patient environment and service attributes, which relate to manpower, patient care and accessibility and effectiveness of service. Process criteria include the professional aspects of nursing care, relating to knowledge and quality of care. Outcome criteria include health and wellness, and good and poor outcomes, which can be incorporated into critical events.

Standards and criteria

Standards are agreed statements of acceptable, observable, achievable and measurable levels of performance. They may also be called policy statements that specify aims. In healthcare, they relate to the quality of care relevant to the needs of the population and healthcare staff. Standards may be set nationally (for example, cervical screening targets), as a district policy (such as infection control policy relevant to the health of a specific population), or locally (specific to a general practice).

Grol (1993) has developed guidelines for quality in general practice. Although aimed at doctors the guidelines are relevant to the nurses who may be delegated the task of assuring quality in one form or another. He emphasises the need for teamwork, planning, consensus and scientific validity when developing guidelines.

Criteria are the descriptive statements, or steps, of how the standard will be met, and must be specific, clear, achievable and clinically sound (Box 2.3). Although most standards are related to actual healthcare, there must also be standards or policy statements on all aspects of general practice management. The practice charter may encompass patient expectations other than health.

Although it is preferable to state that *all* patients should be reviewed annually, a more realistic standard has been set. This can be reviewed following an audit.

Box 2.3   Example of standard and criteria in general practice

Standard: 90% of patients receiving thyroxine will be reviewed and have their blood levels assessed at least annually.

Rationale: To ensure patients receive therapeutic levels of medication.

Criteria: Identify all patients receiving thyroxine – from repeat medication or via disease register

Check date of last blood test for thyroid stimulating hormone (TSH) and/or T4

If not recorded in past 12 months, recall for blood test

Assess concordance with current medication

Determine whether or not the patient is symptomatic

Ensure patient is aware of process for receiving blood results, and advise of annual recall

Annual recall implemented through manual or computer system.

Activity 2.4

Consider the standard and criteria in Box 2.3, and modify to meet the needs of your practice for one aspect of healthcare. For example, how many mental health patients have had a physical health review in the past twelve months?

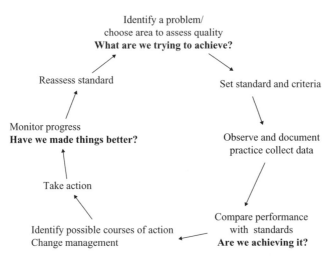

Figure 2.5   An audit cycle.

Audit

Clinical audit was integrated into clinical governance systems (Department of Health 1997) and was stated by the UK Central Council for Nursing Midwifery and Health Visiting (UKCC) to be the business of every registered practitioner (UKCC 2001). Clinical audit is a process of improving patient care through the regular review of care against clear standards, and the implementation of change (Collis 2006; National Institute for Clinical Excellence 2002). A simple audit cycle is shown in Figure 2.5.

Clinical governance improvements must be continuous, and should be viewed as a cyclical process (Collis 2006). Any member of the practice team can undertake audit. The chief source of information for measuring quality outcome is the medical records, which should be fully completed and contemporaneous. Computerised disease registers make this task simpler, as data can be readily accessed for audit purposes, if correctly inputted to the system. Audit will identify areas of action for improvement. In the example in Box 2.3 a policy can be implemented to ensure that all patients who require thyroxine receive a therapeutic dose. Graham (2002) discusses the use of technology to aid audit in the context of risk management.

Excellent practice will motivate the staff to continue to deliver a high level of quality care. However, a deficiency highlighted from an audit should not be viewed negatively, but as a positive outcome. This may result in continuing education for medical and nursing staff and improved effectiveness within the practice team.

Audit need not be a complicated exercise. It is also a tool for coordinating and promoting action on clinical effectiveness (Starey 2003). For example, the quality and effectiveness of minor surgery in general practice may be assessed through documenting the level of post-surgical wound infection (Edwards 1996). The action plan will depend on the level of wound infection noted. No audit will benefit patient care or staff development if staff are not committed to implement recommended changes. Remember that patient safety is a key strand of clinical governance (Donaldson 2004).

Activity 2.5

Use the model in Figure 2.5 to identify an area of care within your practice to develop a quality service. Choose an area you have not examined before.

Patient and staff satisfaction

Customers are said to judge quality by comparing the service they receive against expectations of what they should receive, although their views may be subjective (Ranade 1994). Patient satisfaction may be considered desirable, but a personality clash between patient and health professional may adversely affect this outcome.

Sale (1996) suggests measuring quality of care retrospectively by inviting the patient to discuss their experiences in a post-care interview, which may be structured, unstructured or semi-structured. Although time-consuming, patient feedback is necessary for a quality assessment process. This could be achieved through patient participation groups, where patients are encouraged to air their views. As perceptions alter over time, assessing and monitoring quality in healthcare requires continuous interaction and feedback from patients and staff at all stages of planning and delivering care.

Concurrent measurement (measurement while the patient is in the nurse's care) is more difficult in general practice as some patients are seen only occasionally. One area that can be observed and modified is the level of information given during the consultation.

The needs of staff should not be overlooked. Job satisfaction will affect their contribution to the running of the practice and general patient care, from patients' reception to exit from the premises. The principles will also apply to staff undertaking home visits.

Quality can be measured through patient satisfaction surveys, documentation, observation and interviewing of staff and patients. Only one method should be chosen to obtain a baseline picture for a procedure. Guidance for undertaking surveys can usually be obtained from the Primary Care Trust or institutes of higher education.

Training

As mentioned, objective measurements highlighting excellent practice may motivate staff, while poor results may indicate training needs. The results might suggest that the whole team requires some level of training. For example, a high level of inadequate cervical smears indicates the need for further training for relevant staff. Nurses should not undertake tasks in which they have not been appropriately trained and their competencies assessed; training alone does not ensure competence. Peer review requires sensitive handling, but should be seen as beneficial both to the practitioner and the patient.

Communication

A clear and well-defined shared vision is essential if people are to work well together. An efficient communication channel will enhance the smooth running of a multi-disciplinary general practice team. Feedback is essential to determine the expectation and needs of staff and patients/clients.

Practice meetings and in-house training may present opportunities for feedback, discussion and action on complaints, for which practices should have a publicised complaints procedure. Positive feedback will motivate staff to continue their quality improvement.

Risk management

Risk assessment is a careful examination of what, in your work, could cause harm to people, so that precautions can be taken to prevent harm (Health and Safety Executive 2006). This can include infection control (storage of hazardous materials), staff safety (alarms in rooms), or patient safety (no sharp edges on cupboards). The Health and Safety Executive has practical guidance on these issues.

Risks to patients can be minimised by ensuring critical event audits are undertaken (Pringle 2004; Starey 2003). This is similar to reflection (see Chapter 9), but concentrates on errors or near miss errors, whether caused by medical or nursing staff, communication errors between disciplines (for example hospital discharges with no documentation) or between staff and patient (for example, when a patient displays aggressive behaviour). As with clinical audit, these critical events should be viewed positively, people should learn from them and move forward. They are not intended to deliver blame. A simple critical event audit design is shown in Figure 2.6. Following completion, this should be discussed at a practice meeting, to share the experience and ensure it does not recur. Note that no names are mentioned.

Date:	Place where incident occurred:
What happened	
Why did it happen	
What action was taken	
How could it have been prevented	

Figure 2.6 An example of a format for completing a critical event report.

Time Management

Healthcare is a diverse and flexible business that does not slot into commercial time management specifications. Time is a precious resource that is constant and irreversible, once lost cannot be regained (Clark 2005), and is a key resource necessary for efficient management (Box 2.4). Improved time management may increase efficiency and effectiveness, increase one's feeling of well-being, and subsequently reduce stress. Perry and Rowe (1993) reported that nurses often fail to achieve time management skills; the nature of the work makes this statement unsurprising. The reader is offered the opportunity to reflect on their time management skills that may result in a more efficient working practice rather than increased effort.

Methods and time are closely linked and are related to money. Parkinson's First Law and the Pareto Principle underpin the whole issue of time management and are frequently quoted in management books (Box 2.5).

The workload of general practice staff is dynamic, changing to meet the demands of regular Department of Health reviews. Is time really a shortage, and inevitable, or could we make better use of available time with good planning? Pritchard, Low and Whalen (1986) refer to Parkinson's Law, suggesting that if a person is overloaded with work it may be because he systematically takes too much time to do a job. This can be applied to all areas of work within general practice. The quality of work is not necessarily

---

Box 2.4   Resources at the disposal of management:

- manpower
- money to pay for manpower and materials
- time
- materials
- methods

Box 2.5

Parkinson's First Law
Work expands to fill the time available for the completion of the task

The Pareto Principle
20% of time determines 80% of production; that is, 20% of effort produces 80% of results

related to the time taken to complete a task. One member of staff may achieve the same result in less time than another. However, patient care often involves subjective assessment and is therefore difficult to quantify. The word routine describes an established course or procedure (Adair 1988b). Routines can become mechanical, inflexible, uninspired and therefore more time consuming. Because they are habitual they tend to escape close scrutiny.

Activity 2.6

Write down instances when you have taken longer to do a task than the time allocated. Make notes on why this may have occurred. Examples may include:(1) insufficient time initially allocated for procedure; (2) completing a more thorough assessment of the patient; (3) undertaking other tasks unrelated to the initial consultation, for example hypertension screening or updating immunisations; and (4) chatting to your patient. List ways in which you could have improved your efficiency and effectiveness.

Good organisation involves planning (Box 2.6), delegation and communication. These issues are closely linked and difficult to separate.

Planning

Torrington and Weightman (1994) offer a simple method of recording and analysing current workload to identify areas where inefficiencies lie. Daily activities are recorded for a specified period, at the end of which the record is analysed to identify time spent on particular activities and to propose specific actions to improve efficiency. Although this may appear to be a time wasting exercise, the record may highlight inappropriate workload or poor delegation. Data is then available to support a request for clerical support, more nursing hours or skill mix.

Box 2.6   Planning

Good planning will help to:

- reduce time pressures
- allow creative time (thinking how to set up a task)
- allow preparatory time for organising resources
- permit productive time, when unscheduled jobs are kept to a minimum and deadlines met.

8.30am	Read mail – bin irrelevant
	Put journals to one side to read
	Save mail to answer at end of shift
	Prepare for day's planned work
8.40am	Start appointments/patient care
10.20am	Tidy treatment area
10.30am	Break
10.40am	Continue patient care
12.00md	Tidy treatment area, check stock/re-order
	Take/make telephone calls
	Liase with other disciplines
	Reply to mail
	General administration/ audit/write standards/read journal/see representatives
1.00pm	Lunch

Figure 2.7 Example of planned time management.

Having identified current working practice, it is essential to have a daily diary (Figure 2.7) and a weekly/annual programme to reduce time pressures and allow time for planning.

Individual health needs are not predictable, and it is therefore difficult to allocate a task a set time limit. Schedule a regular time to plan your activities (Clark 2005). This could be for the day, the week or the next month. If a daily planner is not working well, you may be trying to accomplish too much in a day.

The day should be planned to include time for administrative tasks (Box 2.7). If time is used productively, unscheduled jobs are kept to a minimum and deadlines can be met. The quality of time matters more than the quantity of time.

Deskmanship is a skill to be developed. A desk should be clear of all paper except the specific job in hand (Adair 1988b). This allows concentration on one task at a time, and reduces the frustration and tension that accompanies the feeling of being snowed under. A well-organised desk reduces time spent searching for important papers.

Box 2.7   Administration tasks may include:

- reading and answering mail
- writing referral letters
- liaising with colleagues
- making telephone calls
- seeing representatives
- stocking and ordering
- computer work
- writing aims and objectives/standards/audit
- professional development, for example reading journals.

For efficiency, paper should only be handled once; read and reply, read and file, or read and dispose. Circulars and important articles can be filed systematically for access by the practice team.

If administrative time is double booked with general nursing duties, it may be necessary to liaise with the practice manager to remedy the situation. Only 60% of the day should be programmed. This allows time to deal with unexpected situations or emergencies (crises).

Regular morning, lunch and afternoon breaks should be planned into the day to regenerate staff, who will then work better (Godefroy & Clark 1990).

The development of a proactive approach to health, such as health promotion and research demands planned time. Martin (1995) recommends five tools to help nurses find time for research; make research a priority, collaborate with others, break projects into manageable parts, structure work so that one outcome is research, and identify resources.

Prioritising

All tasks should be prioritised (Box 2.8), but it is essential in prioritising not to procrastinate. Procrastination is described as putting off doing something that should be done intentionally, habitually and reprehensibly (Adair 1988b), and is one of the biggest time wasters (Clark 2005). People procrastinate because they are waiting for the right mood, or waiting for the right time. Resolve not to postpone what is ready to be done today. Deal with mail on a daily basis, reply to letters, read the journals, read and file important circulars and bin the rubbish. Writing standards may also be a task that is deferred. Unfortunately these issues will eventually have to be addressed.

Box 2.8   Prioritising

Must do (top priority) – tasks which must be completed or programmed during the day, for example booked appointments

Should do (medium priority) – time element not so important, for example ordering stocks, liaising with other disciplines, writing standards, audit

Could do today, or defer until tomorrow (low priority) – nonessential activities, for example tidying cupboards

---

Activity 2.7

Consider a normal week. Place your regular tasks in one of the three categories of priority. Note any changes you can make to improve your workload.

Crisis intervention

Emergencies (crises) are a common hazard in general practice. Walk-in casualties require priority care. It is essential to take five minutes to regain one's calm, review the list of tasks and re-evaluate the priorities (Godefroy & Clark, 1990). You can learn from a critical experience and prepare for future crises. You may want to complete a critical incident form for practice discussion (see Figure 2.6). The daily diary should allow time for crisis intervention.

Work overload

Professionals experience stress due to too much work (work overload), whereas other workers are more likely to suffer from insufficient work (work underload) (Blyton, Hassard, Hill & Starkey 1989). Work underload is unlikely to apply to any practice staff in the foreseeable future. The worst offenders for time wasting are often those who seem to be working hardest and longest; they do not manage their time well.

Possible causes of work overload for practice nurses include:

- an increase in practice population – new patient checks
- targets for quality outcome framework indicators (Department of Health 2006b)

- extended role of the nurse, including family planning, chronic disease management, cervical cytology
- anything else the general practitioner wishes to delegate
- covering for colleagues who are sick, on leave or taking study days
- insufficient nursing hours for the practice population.

Effectiveness at work depends on knowing what not to do (Professional Development 1994). A nurse who is asked to do more tasks than one can realistically be expected to complete has the right to say 'no'. Learn to decline with tact and firmness. Flexibility is essential. No one should be a slave to a planned daily programme.

Delegation

Work is usually generated by delegation from above and below (Figure 2.8). The most efficient method of time management is through delegation to the person who will be working at their optimum level; that is, the right person for the task (Godefroy & Clark 1990). Delegation saves time and develops subordinates.

Delegation implies transferring initiative and authority to another person to perform an agreed task (Adair 1988b). The subordinate must have the necessary competence for the role, together with a willingness to accept it. Delegation is not abdication of a role, as some degree of control is still necessary. Delegation is a great motivator. It enriches jobs, improves performance and raises morale.

Time should be spent considering which tasks can be delegated up and down the hierarchy. The ordering of health promotion literature, stock checks and input of computer data can be delegated to non-nursing staff.

It may not be appropriate for untrained staff to weigh patients and undertake urinalysis; these procedures necessitate an understanding of the results. However, unqualified staff can be trained to undertake certain tasks that will

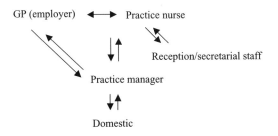

Figure 2.8 Flowchart for delegation.

release time for qualified nurses to utilise their skills (see Chapter 9, skill mix).

Doctors often delegate down to nurses, who should be appropriately trained to undertake specific tasks, to ensure personal professional accountability. Nurses, in their turn, can delegate to healthcare assistants in a skill mix team.

It could be argued that it is inappropriate to delegate child immunisation sessions to practice nurses who have no experience or training in child health. Readers may wish to consider their current position with regard to child immunisation, administration of psychiatric medication and administration of family planning treatments.

Communication and meetings

Good communication allows each team member to know precisely what is required of them. Clear instructions for deadlines prevent misunderstandings. Communication may be oral, written or both. Message books are useful, but must not be used to the exclusion of face-to-face contacts.

It is necessary to spend time to save time. Planning, organising and evaluating teamwork are essential elements of good practice. Regular efficiently chaired practice meetings allow plans to be formulated and evaluated. However, meetings are potential time wasters. An agenda should always be circulated prior to the meeting to increase efficiency. The length of time for the meeting should be specified and adhered to. Multidisciplinary meetings allow feedback of information, and problems and solutions to be discussed.

It can be difficult to ask someone to leave after a meeting, whether formal or informal. Meeting in someone else's office allows the visitor to determine when to leave. Talkative people, including pharmaceutical representatives, are best given an appointment just before lunch. This keeps the meeting short. However, lunch meetings with visitors and colleagues may be a productive use of time.

Nurse meetings are essential for sharing knowledge and planning standards. Time should be allocated for this purpose.

Reducing interruptions

Much of a planned day may be interrupted. These interruptions may classed as 'good' or 'bad', but often cannot be eliminated. A 'good' interruption may be a request to undertake a task for which the nurse is paid, such as wound care or an urgent electrocardiograph. A 'bad' interruption may be an inappropriate telephone call.

Having a set time for taking calls and seeing visitors (pharmaceutical representatives or clinical specialists) can reduce interruptions (Pedler, Burgoyne & Baydell 1986). If a patient or caller has no appointment, it is advisable to set a time limit; for example: 'I have five minutes. Will that do or would you rather fix a time later?'

Incoming telephone calls should be restricted to specified times, such as during a coffee break or at the end of surgery, to avoid interrupting a consultation. Emergency calls are an exception; all staff should be aware of which conditions constitute an urgent call. Details of nonurgent calls could be taken by the reception staff and dealt with at a more appropriate time. Care must be taken by all staff to minimise interruptions.

The worst person for interrupting is yourself (Adair 1988b). This includes breaks for making coffee, dropping one project for another, or stopping work for a chat. These actions must be balanced between time wasting and regenerative breaks.

What about the patient's time?

It must not be forgotten that patients also have to manage their time. Their other commitments may include work, other medical appointments and family or social commitments. Although they like to be seen quickly for their appointments, patients like the doctor or nurse to have plenty of time to listen to their problems (Pritchard et al. 1986). If the nurse runs behind with the appointments, people usually respond well to a simple 'I'm sorry to have kept you waiting' and a thorough consultation. The nurse who regularly falls behind with booked appointments may need to reassess her time management.

Time spent in the initial patient consultation may reduce subsequent consultations. However, for those patients who never seem to want to go home, a pre-arranged telephone call from a colleague can hasten the conclusion of an overlong consultation.

Box 2.9 summarises effective time management in general practice

---

Box 2.9   Methods of achieving effective time management (Edwards 1994)

- Recognition that patients also have to manage their time
- Planning holidays and study leave in advance to spread the workload as evenly as possible
- A daily diary, with specified appointments and duties
- Programming administration time into the day: to include time for professional development
- Appropriate delegation
- Regular breaks to regenerate staff
- Flexibility to deal with crises.

Summary

The importance of a culture and structure that promotes the growth of professional teams, with common aims, is supported by *New World, New Opportunities* (National Health Service Management Executive 1993), which devotes a whole section to team working. It identifies the need for a shared philosophy, the prioritising of aims and health targets and the development of a team/practice management plan. Review of outcomes measured against objectives, through the medium of regular meetings, is highlighted as an essential key to progress. As practice nurses become more autonomous and take on extended roles, the opportunity for moving change forward increases. The organisational culture is unlikely to change, but practice can develop within this arena.

The main purpose of quality assurance activity is to improve or maintain the quality of patient care. This involves all members of the practice team and discussion should be constructive and nonthreatening. Audit should not be viewed simply as a data collection exercise but must be used to improve patient care. Writing standards and undertaking audit are time-consuming processes but are integral to nurses' professional development.

Reflective practice is a positive way that nurses can promote quality healthcare. It must be recognised that patient expectation may differ from that of the health carer, and that one person's perception of quality will vary from another.

It is also important to remember that time is a precious commodity for the patient and the nurse. Pritchard et al. (1986) acknowledge the uncertainty and difficulty of planning in general practice, where staff sickness and crisis management are unavoidable. Training in time management for all staff is essential to improve communication and appreciation of each team member's role.

Improved efficiency through delegation and communication will reduce stress, enhance working conditions and raise morale. Good administrative skills reduce the muddle that makes work and wastes time. Over-preoccupation with time is not an attractive quality. Live one day at a time. You can't change what happened yesterday, but you can make tomorrow better by living well today (Adair 1988b). Quality assurance must be synonymous with quality improvement (Peters 1995).

Key points

- Organisations must have shared goals and objectives
- Communication is the key to good organisation

- Change is inevitable, so become involved from the start
- The primary objective of quality assurance activity is to improve patient care
- Reflective practice is an essential part of professional development in providing quality
- Time is a precious resource, for staff and patients
- Don't be a slave to time

Recommended reading

Handy C (1993) *Understanding Organisations 4th Edn.* Harmondsworth: Penguin.
This book contains an adaptation of a useful self-evaluation questionnaire (Harrison's Inventory), to help you assess the values and styles of your organisation and how these equate with your own.
Kemp N & Richardson E (1990) *Quality Assurance in Nursing Practice.* Oxford: Butterworth-Heinmann.
Miles A & Lugon M (Eds) (1996) *Effective Clinical Practice.* London: Blackwell Science.
Scott CD & Jaffe DT (1990) *Managing Organisational Change.* London: Kogan Page.
This book describes the Transition Grid and the Force-Field Analysis first suggested by Kurt Lewin in 1947. These are simple to apply and provide a practical framework for action.
Van Zwanenberg T & Harrison J (2004) *Clinical Governance in Primary Care 2nd Edn.* Abingdon: Radcliffe Medical Press.

References

Adair J (1988a) *Effective Leadership.* London: Pan Books.
Adair J (1988b) *Effective Time Management. How to Save Time and Spend it Wisely.* London: Pan Books.
Alvaran MSD, Butz A, Larson E (1994) Opinions, knowledge and self reported practices related to infection control among nursing personnel in long term care settings. *American Journal of Infection Control* 22, 367–370.
Armstrong M (2001) *Managing Activities.* Trowbridge: Cromwell Press.
Attree M (1993) An analysis of the concept 'quality' as it relates to contemporary nursing care. *International Journal Nursing Studies* 30(4), 355–369.
Blyton P, Hassard J, Hill S & Starkey K (1989) *Time, Work and Organisation.* London: Routledge.
Broome A (1990) *Managing Change.* London: MacMillan.
Clark D (2005) *Time Management and Leadership.* www.nwlink.com/~donclark/leader/leadtime.html
Collis S (2006) A review of the literature on the nurse role in clinical audit. *Nursing Times* 102(12), 38–40.

Department of Health (1997) *The New NHS; Modern, Dependable.* London: The Stationary Office.

Department of Health (2006a) *Detailed question and answer on 'Practice based commissioning: achieving universal coverage'.* www.dh.gov.uk/PolicyandGuidance/OrganisationPolicy/Commissioning/PracticebasedCommissioning. Accessed 15/4/2006.

Department of Health (2006b) *Quality and Outcomes Frameworks.* London: DOH.

Donabedian A (1988) The quality of care. How can it be assessed? *Journal of American Medical Association* 260(12), 1743–1748.

Donaldson L (2004) Clinical governance: a quality concept. In Van Zwanenberg T & Harrison J (Eds). *Clinical Governance in Primary Care 2nd Edn.* Abingdon: Radcliffe Medical Press.

Drucker P (1974) New templates for today's organisations. In Buchanan DA & Huczynski AA (Eds). *Organizational Behaviour: An Introductory Text.* Hemel Hempstead: Prentice Hall.

Edwards M (1994) Time to go home. *Practice Nursing* 22Mar–4Apr, 20–22.

Edwards M (1996) Assessing quality of general practice care. *Practice Nurse* 12(1), 33–35,37.

Girou E, Loyeau S, Legrand P, Oppein F & Brun-Boisson C (2002) Efficacy of hand rubbing with alcohol based solution versus standard hand washing with antiseptic soap: a randomised trial. *British Medical Journal* 325, 362.

Godefroy C & Clark J (1990) *The Complete Time Management System.* London: Judy Piatkus.

Graham D (2002) Risk management. In Simpson L & Robinson P (Eds). *e-Clinical Governance. A Guide for Primary Care.* Abingdon: Radcliffe Medical Press.

Grol R (1993) Development of guidelines for general practice. *British Journal of General Practice* 43, 146–151.

Handy C (1991) *The Age of Unreason 2nd Edn.* London: Business Ltd.

Handy C (1993) *Understanding Organisations 4th Edn.* Harmondsworth: Penguin.

Health and Safety Executive (2006) *Risk management – practical guidance.* www.hse.gov.uk/risk/practice.htm Accessed 16/4/2006.

Kanter RM (1983) *The Change Masters: Corporate Entrepreneurs at Work.* London: George Allen & Unwin.

King N & Anderson N (2002) *Managing Innovation and Change: A Critical Guide for Organizations.* London: International Thomson Business Press.

Kotter JP & Schleslinger LA (1979) Choosing strategies for change. In Stoner JA & Freeman RE (Eds). *Management.* Englewood Cliffs, NJ: Prentice Hall p 370.

Lewin K (1951) *Field Theory in Social Science: Selected Theoretical Papers.* New York: Harper and Row.

Macgregor Burns J (1978) *Leadership.* New York: Harper and Row.

Martin PA (1995) Ask an expert. Finding time for research. *Applied Nursing Research* 8(3), 151–153.

Murray M (2000) *Ten Commandments.* Presentation at the European Conference on Mental Health Promotion. Birmingham.

Naikoba S & Hayward A (2001) The effectiveness of interventions aimed at increasing hand washing in health care workers – a systematic review. *Journal of Hospital Infection* 47, 173–180.

National Health Service Management Executive (1993) *New World, New Opportunities: Nursing in Primary Health Care.* London: NHSME.

National Institute for Clinical Excellence (2002) *Principles for Best Practice in Clinical Audit.* Oxford: Radcliffe Medical Press.

National Patient Safety Agency (2004) *Clean Your Hands Campaign: The Economic Case.* London: NPSA.

Nursing and Midwifery Council (2004) *The Code of Professional Conduct: Standards for Conduct, Performance and Ethics.* London: NMC.

Ojajarvi J (2003) Alcohol hand rubs v soap. *British Medical Journal* 326, 50.

Ojajarvi J, Makela P & Rantasalo I (1977) Failure of hand disinfection with frequent hand washing: a need for profiled studies. *Journal of Hygiene* 79, 107–119.

Pedler M, Burgoyne J & Baydell T (1986) *Manager's Guide to Self-development.* Maidenhead: McGraw-Hill.

Perry A & Rowe M (1993) Beating time. *Nursing Times* 89(13), 32–34.

Peters DA (1995) Outcomes: The mainstay of a framework for quality care. *Journal of Nursing Care Quality* 10(1), 61–69.

Pringle, M (2004) Significant event auditing. In Van Zwanenberg T & Harrison J (Eds). *Clinical Governance in Primary Care 2nd Edn.* Abingdon: Radcliffe Medical Press.

Pritchard P, Low K & Whalen M (1986) *Management in General Practice.* Oxford: Oxford University Press.

Professional Development (1994) Time management. Revision notes. *Nursing Times* 90(20), Unit 6, Part3/3, p 10

Ranade W (1994) *A Future for the NHS? Health Care in the 1990s.* London: Longman.

Royal College of Nursing (2003) *Clinical Governance: an RCN Resource Guide.* London: RCN.

Sale D (1996) *Quality Assurance. For Nurses and Other Members of the Health Care Team 2nd Edn.* Basingstoke: Macmillan.

Schein EH (1986) *Organisational Culture and Leadership.* San Francisco, CA: Jossey Bass.

Simpson, L (2002) Concepts in clinical governance. In Simpson L & Robinson P (Eds). *e-Clinical Governance. A Guide for Primary Care.* Abingdon: Radcliffe Medical Press.

Starey, N. (2003) *What is clinical governance.* www.evidence-based-medicine.co.uk Accessed 15/4/2006.

Strauss S, Stephen, H, Sonnex C & Gray J (2003) Contamination of environmental surfaces by genital human papillomavirus (HPV): a follow up study. *Sexually Transmitted Infections* 79(5), 426–427.

Strong P & Robinson J (1990) *The NHS under New Management.* Milton Keynes: Open University Press.

Sullivan E & Decker P (1997) *Effective Leadership and Management in Nursing 4th Edn.* Harlow: Addison-Wesley.

Tiffany C & Lutjens L (1998) *Planned Change Theories for Nursing.* London: Sage.

Torrington D & Weightman J (1989) *Effective Management: People and Organisations.* London: Prentice Hall.

Torrington D & Weightman J (1994) *Effective Management 2nd Edn.* London: Prentice Hall.

Townsend P, Whitehead M & Davidson N (1992) *Inequalities of Health.* London: Penguin.

United Kingdom Central Council for Nursing Midwifery and Health Visiting (2001) *Professional Self-Regulation and Clinical Governance.* London: UKCC.

Van Zwanenberg T & Harrison J (2004) *Clinical Governance in Primary Care 2nd Edn.* Abingdon: Radcliffe Medical Press.

Wall D, Gerada C, Conlon M, Ombler-Spain S & Warner L (2006) Supporting clinical governance in primary care. *Clinical Governance: an International Journal* 11(1), 30–38.

Workforce and Development Leadership Working Group (2000) *Workforce and Development – Embodying Leadership in the NHS.* London: NHS.

Chapter 3

Infection Control

Mandy Beaumont and Chris Baldwin

The National Audit Office (2000) reported that about 5,000 deaths a year are attributable to healthcare associated infections (HCAIs). Patients no longer stay in hospital as long as they used to and many have procedures that would once have been undertaken in hospital, but that are now performed in the community. Hence healthcare associated infections are every member of the healthcare staff's responsibility, not just that of hospital staff. There has been a flurry of new guidance from the Department of Health and the National Patient Safety Agency and this chapter will explore some of these in the context of the community and GP setting.

Infection control should be a routine part of the practice nurse's role. This chapter has been updated to help practice nurses assess their current practice and identify areas in which improvement can be made. In addition, a brief overview of some of the more common healthcare acquired infections will be given.

It is accepted that changing a practice routine and obtaining the resources to change policy can be very difficult (see Chapter 2, Change management). Small changes will lead to an overall improvement in infection control; many small changes will make a significant difference. Readers who currently meet all the recommendations are to be commended.

'Does not the popular idea of infection involve that people should take greater care of themselves than the patient? That for instance it is safer to not to be too much with the patient, not to attend too much to his wants? Perhaps the best illustration of the utter absurdity of this view of duty in attending on infectious diseases is afforded by what was very recently the practice, if it is not so even now, . . . in which the plague-patient used to be condemned to the horrors of filth, overcrowding and want of ventilation, while the medical attendant was ordered to examine the patient's tongue through an opera glass and to toss him a lancet to open his own abscess with, . . . True nursing ignores infection except to prevent it . . . Wise and

The Informed Practice Nurse, Edwards, M. (2008), Chichester: Wiley.

humane management of the patient is the best safeguard against infection'
(Nightingale 1859).

Introduction

Communicability is a factor that differentiates infection from noninfectious
diseases. The transmission of pathogenic organisms to other people, directly
or indirectly, may lead to an outbreak of infection. Many infections are preventable by hygiene measures, by vaccines or by wise use of drugs
(chemoprophylaxis).

Infection control has been practised in a variety of fragmented forms since
1850 when Semmelweiss noted varying mortality rates from puerperal sepsis
in deliveries undertaken by different staff groups. It is a system of methods
by which patients are protected from infection (Ayliffe, Lowbury, Geddes &
Williams 1992). It is fundamental to the provision of a safe environment and
quality care for patients. The EPIC group (Pratt et al. 2007) reiterated the
standard infection control precautions that need to be applied by *all* healthcare practitioners to the care of *all* patients. These shall be discussed in
further detail later in the chapter.

There is past evidence that the standard of infection control knowledge
among general nurses is poor (Gould 1995). Studies have also shown that
the provision for good infection control in general practice is poor (Foy,
Gallagher & Rhodes 1990; Hoffman, Cooke & Larkin 1988). There is no recent
evidence to contradict these studies.

With the shift in emphasis from secondary to primary healthcare provision, and with increasing numbers of minor surgical interventions, it is
essential that infection control becomes a priority within the general practice
arena. A Primary Care Trust (PCT) commissioning service from a nonNHS
body should satisfy itself that its contractors have appropriate systems in
place to keep patients, staff and visitors safe from HCAIs (Department of
Health 2006a).

There have been successes in the control of communicable disease in the
past century, although credit is due more to improvements in nutrition and
living conditions than immunisation and antibiotics. Factors that have influenced how infections have developed since the mid-1970s are summarised
in Box 3.1.

Pathology of infection

Disease due to infection is the result of the interaction between microorganisms and the defence mechanisms of the body. Infection occurs when the
microorganisms gain the upper hand.

Box 3.1   Factors influencing patterns of infection

- Microbial resistance
- Immune suppression
- Foreign travel
- Sexual behaviour
- Illicit drug usage
- New and emerging diseases
- Changes in animal husbandry
- Food production
- Availability/uptake of vaccines
- Improved standard of living.

Source and spread

Infection that may originate from the patient (autogenous) is usually from the skin, nasopharynx or bowel. Outside (exogenous) sources include another person who is suffering from infection or carrying pathogenic microorganisms; and from contaminated equipment or the environment itself. Carriers are usually healthy and may harbour the organism in their throat (for example diphtheria), bowel (for example salmonella) or blood (for example hepatitis B).

Reservoirs of infection other than humans include:

- Water – Legionnaires disease (only when water aerosolised)
- Milk – salmonella food poisoning
- Food – campylobacter food poisoning (mainly poultry)
- Animals – tuberculosis (mainly cattle)
- Birds – psittacosis
- Soil and water – cryptosporidiosis.

Definitions

The following list gives definitions of some of the common terms associated with infections.

- *Colonisation* – where organisms are present but there is no host reaction to their presence. Analysis of microbiological swabs is the only way of identifying whether a patient is colonised with an organism.
- *Infection* – invasion and multiplication of microorganisms in body tissues causing local cellulitis. The classic signs of infection are redness; heat; pain; swelling; and pus.

- *Incubation period* – the time between the invasion of the tissues by pathogens and the appearance of clinical features of acute illness.
- *Period of infectivity* – the period of time during which the patient is infectious to others.
- *Bacteraemia* – the presence of living microorganisms in the blood, which can occur in people without causing symptoms.
- *Septicaemia* – occurs when organisms enter the bloodstream, actively multiply and produce toxins. Organisms causing septicaemia may originate from one of the areas of the body that are normally colonised by microorganisms, for example large bowel and genital tract, or may enter the bloodstream from another part of the body that is already infected such as the bladder.
- *Toxaemia* – a concentration of bacterial toxins in the blood.
- *Acute illness* – the stage at which the disease reaches its full intensity.

Standard precautions

The Department of Health (UK Health Departments 1990) recommended that all healthcare workers should adopt 'universal precautions' when caring for patients. These have been updated since then and are now referred to as 'Standard Precautions' (Box 3.2).

The Health Act 2006 suggests that standard precautions mainly involve hand hygiene and the use of personal protective equipment (Department of Health 2006a). Sharps disposal, inoculation injury guidelines, ensuring a clean environment and appropriate decontamination and sterilisation of

---

Box 3.2   Standard precautions (Infection Control Nurses Association 2003; Royal College of Nursing 2005)

1. Cover all cuts and abrasions and lesions with a waterproof dressing
2. Maintain hand hygiene
3. Maintain cleanliness of patient's environment
4. Use personal protective equipment when handling blood and body fluids
5. Dispose of contaminated waste safely, including laundry
6. Undertake appropriate decontamination of equipment
7. Ensure management of exposure to blood or body fluids
8. Isolate patients with a known or suspected infection.

equipment, as well as prudent antibiotic prescribing, are listed as Clinical Care Protocols and are recognised as being essential in the control of infection.

Hand hygiene

As hand washing has been described as the single most important control measure in the control of infection (Ayliffe et al. 1992), we shall consider it first. Hand hygiene describes a process that removes potentially pathogenic organisms from the hands, the aim of which is to prevent the hands becoming a vehicle for cross-infection.

In order to reduce the transmission of infection it is vital that the hands of the healthcare worker are washed before and after each patient contact (Department of Health 2006b) and that the hand-washing technique is of a high standard. In order to prevent the spread of infection, practice nurses need to be able to challenge their own hand-washing technique and that of their colleagues. Types of hand hygiene are summarized in Table 3.1.

The importance of hand hygiene as a means of preventing cross-infection should be the first task the student nurse learns. However, despite knowledge, training and continuing education, nurses do not always wash their hands as often, or as well, as they should.

Taylor (1978) found that some nurses thought there was no risk of cross-infection if they had not touched a soiled object or their hands did not look dirty. It is hoped that, if Taylor's research were conducted in 2008, the results might be a little more favourable and there would have been an improvement in the hand-washing technique of all healthcare workers.

Table 3.1 Types of hand hygiene

Type	Materials	When used
Social	Soap and water	After visiting the toilet and before starting work, going home or attending to the next patient
Hygienic	Medicated soap, e.g. chlorhexidine	Before aseptic technique and after contact with an infected patient
Surgical	Chlorhexidine, povidone iodine	Prior to surgical intervention to remove transient organisms and a substantial number of resident organisms

Resources

The resources used for hand washing must not create a cross-infection hazard. Bowell (1992) states that poorly cleaned and maintained hand basins and soap dispensers may create a cross-infection risk. Available resources must be well maintained and, if broken, damaged, or the practice nurse considers that they are a cross-infection risk, the equipment must be replaced. Advice about replacing equipment should be sought from a local infection control advisor.

Hand-washing technique

The hand-washing technique described in Box 3.3 is based on a procedure described by Ayliffe et al. in 1992 and is recommended as the most effective way of decontaminating hands. Box 3.4 describes the procedure prior to minor surgery; there might be occasions when the nurse has to remind a doctor of good practice.

Box 3.3   Recommended six-stage hand-washing technique (Ayliffe et al. 1992)

Sufficient soap should be applied to the hands to obtain a good lather. Hand-washing or disinfecting technique, regardless of the product selected, must ensure that no area of the skin surface of the hand is missed during the procedure.

Rub the hands

1. palm to palm
2. right palm over left dorsum, left palm over right dorsum
3. palm to palm finger interlaced
4. backs of fingers to opposing palms with fingers interlocked
5. rotating rubbing of right thumb clasped in left palm and vice versa
6. rotational rubbing backwards and forwards with the clasped fingers of right hand in left palm and vice versa.

Rinsing and drying hands

Following the application of the soap the hands should be thoroughly rinsed under warm running water for a further 10–15 seconds and dried using a disposable paper towel.

Box 3.4   Hand-washing requirements for minor surgery:

- The hand washing sink should be fitted with an elbow-operated mixer tap.
- There must be a supply of soap and disposable paper towels in dispensers next to the sink.
- There must be a foot-operated pedal bin for the safe disposal of used paper towels.
- If nailbrushes are used, they should be single use and sterile; repeated scrubbing with nailbrushes will damage the skin and may be associated with an increase in the number of resident bacteria.
- Before the first surgical case, the hands and forearms should be washed thoroughly with soap and water for two minutes.

Note that:

- Antiseptic detergent hand-wash preparations are usually chlorhexidine or iodine based.
- Surgical hand disinfection should be carried out prior to performing any minor surgery.

Hands should be washed:

Before
- patient contact
- aseptic technique
- handling food or medicines.

After
- patient contact
- removing protective clothing
- handling blood or body fluids
- handling waste.

Alcohol hand rub

Alcohol hand rub can assist in facilitating hand hygiene in as much as it can be used at the point at which staff deliver care (Department of Health 2006b, 2006c). Staff should be aware, however, that alcohol hand rub is not thought to be effective against some organisms such as *Clostridium difficile*.

The six-stage technique in Box 3.3 is appropriate for the application of alcohol hand rub, which can be used when there is no access to a sink.

In the primary healthcare setting there are many procedures undertaken in one area. Ideally a separate room would be allocated specifically for minor surgery, but in practice it is uncommon for practice premises to allow separate clinical rooms for minor surgery, health promotion and treatment room tasks. It is therefore vital that hand-cleansing facilities are conveniently located throughout the clinical area.

Personal protective equipment (PPE)

In the past, healthcare workers have been encouraged to reduce the use of protective clothing, in the belief that it demonstrated a barrier to communication. However, with the advent of Human Immunodeficiency Virus (HIV) in the early 1980s the use of protective clothing has become common practice for nurses in the clinical area. Plastic aprons and disposable gloves should be worn when the practitioner expects contact with blood or body fluids (Health and Safety Executive 1994). PPE is designed to provide a barrier between the patient and the healthcare worker that can be removed before contact with other patients. Its use will reduce the risk of transmission of microorganisms from one person to another. It is not intended that wearing gloves should replace hand washing: they should be employed in addition to thorough hand decontamination. Box 3.5 offers guidance for glove use.

The decision to wear gloves rests with the practitioner. The practice nurse has to make an informed choice through risk assessment about glove usage, remembering that the protection of both client and healthcare worker is vital.

Box 3.5   Guidance for glove use

Gloves should be used:

- to prevent hands becoming contaminated
- to prevent the transfer of organisms already present on the skin and to minimise cross-infection, thereby protecting the nurse and the client
- to protect the user while handling infectious material, such as blood, faeces and urine
- to protect the client from transient microorganisms.

Sharps disposal

A report by the Health Protection Agency explored the ongoing risks to healthcare staff of sharps injury (Health Protection Agency 2005a). Of the 2,140 sharps injuries reported during a seven-year period there were nine hepatitis C sero-conversions. All staff in the practice must be aware of the safe management of needles and what follow up is required should they sustain an injury. Needles should not be re-sheathed. The syringe and needle should be discarded as one unit into a recommended sharps container, which must comply with BS7320 and UN3291; sharps must never be left to be disposed of by someone else. Sharps containers should be sealed and labelled with the name of the practice and discarded when they are no more than three-quarter full (they should **never** be placed in a yellow bag). A registered company must finally incinerate all sharps. Sharps boxes in use must be out of the reach of patients and children.

Inoculation injury and mucous membrane splash guidelines are outlined in Box 3.6.

(For more detailed information about management of sharps injuries and post-exposure prophylaxis see Department of Health 2004.)

Minor surgery within general practice

Minor surgical operations have been part of general practice for many years and are now an enhanced service within the general practitioner GMS contract (National Health Service Confederation/BMA 2003). It is now part of everyday life for the practice nurse, and the role in minor surgery is vital. The outcome of the procedure depends on the skill of the doctor and the nursing support, alongside the implementation of good infection control procedures.

The clinical room

Clean and dirty areas should be clearly defined to reduce the risk of cross-infection. Recommendations for cleaning clinical areas are listed in Table 3.2. All surfaces should be impermeable and easy to clean.

Appropriate protective clothing, such as plastic aprons and household gloves, should be worn during all cleaning procedures. Cleaning equipment such as mops should be used only in the clinical areas. Cloths should be disposable. Colour coding is essential in ensuring that equipment is not used in other areas of practice (National Patient Safety Agency 2006) (see Table 3.3).

Box 3.6   Inoculation injury guidelines

First aid

Inoculation injury	Mucous membrane splash, e.g. mouth, eyes
Stop what you are doing and attend to the injury	Stop what you are doing and attend to the splashed mucous membranes
Bleed the area	Rinse the area thoroughly with copious amounts of warm water
Always wash the injured area with soap and running, warm water	
Cover with a waterproof plaster	
Report the incident to line manager	

Report the incident

A record of the whole incident must be made and kept. This should include the names of the people involved.

Further action required *(This is also relevant if the injured party is a member of the general public)*

It will be necessary to take blood from the injured person, which will be sent for storage only.

It is necessary to request blood from the source patient and this should be tested for HIV, Hepatitis B and C virus following informed consent and counselling. It is not appropriate for the injured party to approach the source asking them to have their blood tested but should be done by an independent clinician.

Contact your occupational health advisor or the Infection Control Team within the PCT or Consultant in Communicable Disease Control based within the Health Protection Unit for detailed information on local policy.

NB Keep an up-to-date protocol in your infection control folder.

Table 3.2   Colour coding for cleaning equipment in general practice (NPSA 2006)

Colour	Area
Red	Toilets, basins and bathroom floors
Blue	General areas including offices and basins in public areas
Green	Kitchens

Table 3.3   Infection control in the clinical room (Infection Control Nurses Association 2003)

Fixture	Type	Method of cleaning
Hand wash basins	Basin should have smooth easy-to-clean surfaces. Overflows are not recommended and the sink should not have a plug. There should be elbow-operated or sensor-activated mixer taps	Daily cleaning with detergent and water
Paper towels and liquid soap	Paper towels and liquid soap should be available at the sink in dispensers. Nailbrushes must be single use only	Wipe dispensers daily with water and detergent to prevent build up of dust
Decontamination sink	This should be allocated in a dirty utility room or designated dirty area in the clinical area and used solely for the purpose of washing equipment. There should be a plug in the sink, elbow-operated taps and a draining board	
Floors	Vinyl non-slip with welded seams	Clean daily at the end of each day or session using detergent and water
Walls	Must be dry and free from cracks. Painted with oil-based paint to withstand regular cleaning. Areas behind sinks and work surfaces should be protected with plastic or stainless steel splash backs. Tiling not recommended for new builds	Cleaned on a six-monthly basis or when visibly soiled

Table 3.3   *Continued*

Fixture	Type	Method of cleaning
Work surfaces	These should be smooth and impervious, and able to withstand chemical disinfectants. They should be roll edged and preferably made from stainless steel	Wiped down using detergent and water after each procedure and after each session
Radiators	Painted with oil-based paint	Cleaned on a six-monthly basis or when visibly soiled
Storage facilities	Cupboards with lockable doors should be used as storage. Open shelving is not recommended because of the difficulty in cleaning and the potential for contamination of products	Doors should be wiped down daily with water and detergent
Treatment couches	The covering must be intact and impervious. A disposable paper cover should be used for each patient	These should be washed down after each procedure and at the end of each session with detergent and water
Examination lights	Easy to clean to prevent build up of dust	Clean using a damp cloth soaked in water and detergent at the end of each session
Mechanical ventilation, such as electric extractor fan	Easy to clean	Inspect on a monthly basis and clean on a three-monthly basis to prevent the build up of dust
Suction tubing	Should be disposable	Disposable
Suction jar	Should have a disposable liner	Disposable liner. Filters to be changed in line with manufacturers instructions.
Cubicle curtains	Curtains should be able to withstand a hot wash	Cleaned every six months or when visibly soiled

Equipment

Disposable paper sheeting should be used for examination and operating couches. Blankets and sheets and pillowcases should not be used.

Preparing the patient

The aim of disinfecting the skin sites prior to surgery is to remove and reduce the number of resident bacteria and reduce the risk of endogenous infection.

The preparation product used should be fast acting and have a prolonged antibacterial effect, although skin reactions may occur with some products. It may be necessary to do a skin test first to check for allergy. The skin cleansing solution should be applied liberally to the site and surrounding area, and then allowed to dry. Skin disinfection should be carried out immediately prior to surgery. Shaving is not recommended because this has been found to increase the risk of infection.

Personal protective equipment

The nurse assisting in minor surgical procedures should wear a disposable plastic apron. Latex free sterile gloves should be used for any procedure involving contact with normally sterile areas of the body. Gloves and aprons should be disposed of as clinical waste.

Waste

Disposal of waste from general practice is guided by the best practice principles of HTM07-01 safe management of healthcare waste (Department of Health 2006d). This introduces new methodology for identifying infectious and medicinal waste that complies with regulations of health and safety, transport and waste. The clinical waste classification of groups A–E waste has been superseded by this guidance and there is a revised colour-coded best practice waste segregation and packaging system (see Box 3.7). Grade E waste for instance is now referred to as offensive/hygiene waste (sanitary protection, nappies and incontinence) and is classified noninfectious but does require appropriate segregation in yellow bags with a black stripe on them. Infectious waste, for example blood-stained dressings, should be placed in orange bags in foot/knee operated waste bins. Waste bags should be removed at the end of each session or day and placed in a designated holding area.

Management of healthcare waste is complex and the practice nurse/practice manager would be advised to check with their local PCT or infection control adviser as to whether they are complying with current guidance.

Protection of staff and patients

Patient safety must be safeguarded at all times. The immunisation of staff against hepatitis B is essential, and all healthcare staff must comply with Department of Health (2006e) guidelines on hepatitis B.

Box 3.7   Revised colour-coded best practice waste segregation for waste produced in general practice (Department of Health 2006d)

Yellow bag with red line	Infectious waste contaminated with cytotoxic material/cytotoxic medicines
Yellow sharps bin with red top	Sharps contaminated with cytotoxic material or cytotoxic medicines
Yellow sharps bin with yellow top	Partially discharged sharps not contaminated with cytotoxic material
Sharps box with orange top	Sharps not contaminated with medicinal products or fully discharged sharps with products other than cytotoxic material
Orange bag	Infectious and potentially infectious waste
Yellow bag with black stripe	Offensive hygiene waste
Black bag	Domestic waste

Disinfection

The decontamination of equipment between patients, especially where there is a high risk of spread of infection, is the responsibility of the practice nurse. Nonadherence to safe practice will jeopardise the standard of care delivered to the patient and will therefore be a direct violation of the NMC Code of Conduct for nurses (see Chapter 1).

All disinfectants are potentially hazardous and must be used with caution. For example, hypochlorites corrode metals and bleach fabrics. Hypochlorite concentration is measured in parts per million (ppm) available chlorine. It is recommended that spills of blood be disinfected by cleaning with 10,000 ppm available chlorine and that for other purposes 1,000 ppm available chlorine is sufficient. However, as suggested above, there are many surfaces that will be damaged by the use of hypochlorite. All disinfectants should be assessed for risk under the requirement of the Control of Substances Hazardous to Health (COSHH) regulations 1994 (Health and Safety Executive 1994) and stored in a locked cupboard accordingly. Liquid bleach, which is less safe and less convenient than hypochlorite, should be stored

Table 3.4 Spillage guidelines

Type	Method
Urine	Clean with general purpose detergent and dry area thoroughly
Faeces/vomit	Wipe up spillages with disposable paper towels. Clean the area using general purpose detergent and dry thoroughly
Blood	Use chlorine granules to soak up the blood and remove granules with paper towel or scoop. Wash the area with general purpose detergent

in a cool, dark place and used within six months. Fresh solutions of cleaning agents should be made up daily as required.

Any spillage must be cleaned up as soon as possible. Always wear an apron and disposable gloves before handling any body fluids. Spillages of blood and body fluids should be dealt with as described in Table 3.4.

Care should be taken to ensure chlorine granules are not used on urine spills because of the potential reaction between the two fluids that may release a chlorine gas.

A spillage kit can be bought commercially or should be made up to include chorine granules, clinical waste bag, disposable gloves, goggles, an apron and a scoop. All staff should be aware of how to use the spillage kit appropriately.

Sterilisation

Benchtop sterilisers are no longer regarded as the most appropriate way to sterilise medical equipment within general practice. Where possible decontamination should always be carried out in dedicated facilities for example:

- Endoscopes – endoscopy suite
- Surgical instruments – sterile services

Alternatively the practice should consider using disposable equipment.

It is important to understand the processes leading to sterilisation:

Decontamination: A combination of processes which removes or destroys contamination so that infectious agents or other contaminants cannot reach a susceptible site in sufficient quantities to initiate infection or other harmful response.

Cleaning: Physical removal of organic matter and infectious agents.

Table 3.5 Recommendations for cleaning/sterilising equipment

Risk	Application	Recommendation
High	Items in contact with a break in the skin or mucous membrane, or introduced into a sterile part of the body; for example surgical instruments	These instruments must be sterile at the point of use
Intermediate	Items in contact with intact skin, mucous membranes or body fluids, particularly after use on infected patients or prior to use on immunocompromised patients, e.g. examination specula	Must be sterilised or disposed of after use. Consider the use of single use items. Single use items must not be reprocessed
Low	Items in contact with intact skin or mucous membranes or not in contact with the patient, example, e.g. thermometers, auroscope probes, hard surfaces	Clean with general purpose detergent and dry thoroughly. Alternatively some equipment has disposable covers which should be changed between patients, e.g. disposable thermometer covers

Disinfection: Reduction in viable infectious agents.
Sterilisation: Render an object free from all viable infectious agents.

Table 3.5 lists the recommendations for cleaning and sterilising equipment.

Control of Substances Hazardous to Health (COSHH)

The 1988 COSHH regulations, updated in 1994 (Health and Safety Executive 1994), cover substances that can cause ill health to either workers or others exposed to those substances. These include those substances that:

- are used at work: chemicals such as cleaning materials
- arise from work: fumes and waste products
- occur naturally: microorganisms

COSHH regulations require that hazardous substances are identified in the work place and procedures implemented to protect staff and visitors from the workplace.

Identification

It is important to identify all materials within the work place that must comply with COSHH regulations. In the case of chemicals their warning label can identify these.

Assessment

It is important that the hazard and the risk are assessed (see Chapter 2, Management/risk management). Chemicals, for example, may be flammable or harmful if swallowed, and a risk assessment needs to be completed and recorded, which identifies the hazard of each chemical used in the practice.

The hazard is the potential of the substance to cause harm, and the risk is the likelihood that it will cause harm in the actual circumstances of use. For example, there can be a risk from a material that is not particularly hazardous if it is used inappropriately and carelessly, whereas the risk of being harmed by a hazardous substance can be very slight if proper precautions are taken.

Control measures

To prevent exposure, the harmful substance should be substituted, where possible, by a non-harmful substance. The process should be enclosed (controlled) by identifying systems of safe working and the use of PPE.

Monitor

Staff working with chemicals that have been identified as hazardous to health may need occupational health check ups and follow-up. Within general practice, it is unlikely that there will be any chemicals that fall into this category unless staff are dealing with Gluteraldehyde, which is not recommended for routine use.

Maintain

A programme of continuing training and education should be available for all staff within general practice. This should include information for non-clinical staff in the handling of specimens of blood or other body fluid where microorganisms may be present.

Inform

Staff are encouraged to report any problems that they encounter.

Vaccine storage

The cold chain and its maintenance is an important component of any immunisation programme. Immunisation gives rise to immunity, and immunity of the population leads to disease reduction. However, immunity can result only from the use of active and effective vaccines. Adu et al. (1996) describe active and effective vaccines as needing four essential elements within the cold chain in order to sustain potency:

1. Equipment – well-insulated cool boxes, designated well-maintained fridges and a maximum/minimum thermometer
2. Manpower – trained staff
3. Transportation – appropriate vehicles and speed
4. Vaccines – quality of the vaccine at the time of administration.

A break in the cold chain at any of these points has long been associated with a low sero-conversion rate in vaccine programmes.

Guidelines to ensure correct storage of vaccines are taken from the Department of Health (2006e) and listed in Box 3.8.

Check list for the practice nurse

This checklist should be used daily by the appointed responsible person or under their direct supervision.

- Read maximum/minimum thermometer and record temperature. Record what action is taken if outside the recommended temperature range
- Does the fridge need defrosting?
- Warning message is visible 'This refrigerator contains vaccines and should not be switched off'
- Refrigerator is packed safely and not overcrowded. Vaccine packs are not touching the sides of the refrigerator or coming into contact with ice
- Door of refrigerator closes properly
- Vaccine receipts book is up to date. Vaccine type, date and quantity received, batch number, expiry date, number of doses used, number returned to pharmacy, current stock as number of doses.

Box 3.8   Correct storage of vaccines (DH 2006e)

- All vaccines should be stored as recommended by the manufacturer of the vaccine, in order to maintain their potency
- All vaccines should be stored between 2°C and 8°C, protected from light and not allowed to freeze
- Ensure a good stock rotation of the vaccines. Shorter dated vaccines should be put at the front of the fridge to ensure they are used first
- A specialised vaccine fridge should be used – domestic fridges must not be used
- Food, drink and specimens must not be stored in the vaccine fridge
- Vaccines should not touch the side of the fridge or be stored in the door
- Vaccines should not be packed tightly into the fridge. The air must circulate around the fridge for the fridge to operate correctly
- Opening of the fridge door should be kept to a minimum in order to maintain a constant temperature
- Interruption to the electricity supply to the fridge can be prevented by using a switchless socket or by placing a notice on the socket or the fridge stating that the fridge should not be turned off at any time
- Records of regular servicing, defrosting and cleaning should be kept
- Temperatures should be recorded each working day. Calibration of thermometers should checked annually
- Arrangements should be in place for backup facilities to be available in the event of the refrigerator failing or breaking down
- When transporting vaccines the cold chain must be maintained. Vaccines should always be carried in a cool box, ensuring the cool pack does not allow the vaccine to freeze
- Always read the manufacturers' leaflets about reconstitution and stability of reconstituted vaccines. All unused reconstituted vaccines should be disposed of at the end of an immunisation session by sealing in a proper, puncture resistant 'sharps' box (UN-approved BS7320)

Healthcare associated infections

Healthcare associated infections are of great national concern. The following is a summary of key information about organisms that the practice nurse may find useful when dealing with patients who have the infection or are worried they may acquire the infection.

Clostridium difficile

In common with several other developed countries, the number of reported cases of *Clostridium difficile* associated disease (CDAD) in England and Wales has increased dramatically during the past decade (HPA 2005b). The voluntary surveillance (to Public Health Laboratory Services and later the HPA) of CDAD reported 10,039 cases in 1995 and 49,850 cases in 2005. This increase is probably caused by two events, that is an actual increase in the numbers of people being affected and an increase in the number of samples being tested for CDAD following the recommendations made by the National *Clostridium difficile* Standards Group (2003). The number of death certificates mentioning CDAD has risen from 975 deaths in 1999 to 2247 in 2004 reflecting the increasing numbers of infection overall (Office of National Statistics 2006).

The Healthcare Commission (2006) reported an investigation into the outbreaks during 2003–2005 of CDAD at Stoke Mandeville Hospital where over 30 people died as a consequence of the infection. Further recommendations into the management of cases of CDAD were made as a result of this report. A new more and more virulent type of *C. difficile* (027) has been identified recently, which is associated with more deaths, illness and relapses than other strains.

In order to reduce the number of cases of all *C. difficile,* the Department of Health has issued guidance that includes a mandatory surveillance programme of all cases of *C. difficile* isolated in microbiology departments in anyone aged 2 years or over (Chief Medical Officer 2007). Preventative measures are based around prudent antibiotic prescribing and encouraging prescribers to adhere to local policy.

Although patients with symptoms of *C. difficile* are unlikely to attend their GP surgery, staff should be aware about the importance of the following should a symptomatic patient be seen in the surgery:

- Hand hygiene – wash hands with soap and water before and after each patient contact. It is recommended that staff do not use alcohol hand rub if they have been in contact with *C. difficile* as there is a question mark as to its effectiveness
- Enhanced environmental cleaning using chlorine based disinfectants to reduce environmental contamination with *C. difficile* spores
- Use of personal protective equipment.

Some of the questions that the practice nurse may be asked are listed in Box 3.9 with appropriate responses.

Box 3.9   Questions and answers about *Clostridium difficile*

What is **Clostridium difficile** *(C. diff)?*

C. *diff* can be found in the gut as part of the normal bowel flora.

Why does it cause disease?

If the normal bowel flora is disrupted by antibiotic therapy, the C. *diff* can multiply in the absence of other gut flora and take over the gut wall. The C. *diff* produces a toxin and it is this toxin that causes the symptoms.

What are the symptoms of **C. diff** *infection?*

Symptoms caused by C. *diff* vary from diarrhoea to a life-threatening pseudomembraneous colitis with a toxic mega colon. The diarrhoea can be extremely severe and may last for 48 hours or more. This can be particularly debilitating in the elderly. The risk of dehydration is high.

How can it be treated?

Occasionally discontinuing the offending antibiotic therapy is enough to stop the symptoms and allow the bowel to recover. However, many may require specific antibiotics to tackle the C. *diff* infection. Hospitalisation may be required if the infection is particularly severe.

How can the spread of **C. diff** *be avoided in the home setting?*

C. *diff* organisms can contaminate the environment and can survive for long periods in the environment because of its ability to spore. It is essential that the environment of a patient with C. *diff* is kept clean. Lavatory areas should be cleaned with a bleach-based product and where possible the infected person should not share the lavatory with others. Household contacts should be advised about thorough hand hygiene and wearing disposable gloves (e.g. household gloves) when cleaning or handling soiled linen. Laundry should be washed on the hottest setting the linen can tolerate. Soiled incontinence pads should be wrapped thoroughly and disposed of in the usual manner according to local policy.

Meticillin-resistant Staphylococcus aureus

Staphylococcus aureus is a Gram-positive coccus and is present in the normal nasal flora of 30 per cent of individuals and on the perineum in 15 per cent of people. It can be transiently carried on the hands of healthcare staff and can survive well in the environment on skin scales and in dust.

Meticillin-resistant *Staphylococcus aureus* (MRSA) strains were first reported in 1961 and have since been responsible for outbreaks of infection in many parts of the world. Microbiology departments have been reporting isolates of all *Staphylococcus aureus* in blood since 1990. The number of reported cases has risen exponentially from 4,955 in 1990 to 15,136 in 2005, over a third of these in 2005 are MRSA. All MRSA bacteraemias are now reported by Acute Trusts to the Strategic Health Authority on UNIFY via Serious Untoward Incidents, and a ROOT Cause Analysis has to be completed regardless of whether the patient appeared to have acquired the MRSA infection in or outside hospital.

Some of the questions that the practice nurse is likely to be asked are listed in Box 3.10 with appropriate responses.

Panton Valentine Leukocidin Staphylococcus aureus

Panton Valentine Leukocidin (PVL) is a toxic substance produced by some strains of *Staphylococcus aureus* both Meticillin sensitive and resistant (Health Protection Agency PVL Working Group 2006). It is associated with an increased ability of the organism to cause disease. PVL strains of *Staphylococcus aureus* commonly cause soft tissue infections e.g. cellulites or abscesses, boils and carbuncles. On rare occasions they can cause more severe infection, for example septic arthritis, bacteraemia or a severe life-threatening form of pneumonia. People may be colonised with this form of *Staphylococcus aureus* without having infection. However, damage to the skin through cuts and abrasions may lead to infection. Those patients who should be suspected of PVL-*Staphylococcus aureus* are those with a history of recurrent boils or other soft tissue infections, participators in contact sports, military personnel and residents of care homes. At present final UK guidance on the management of PVL-*Staphylococcus aureus* is awaited. Certainly standard infection control procedures are essential in the control of this organism (see Box 3.2 on standard precautions). In some cases a decolonisation regime for the affected person may be recommended and sometimes screening of close contacts may be required.

Extended Spectrum β Lactamase

Extended Spectrum β Lactamase (ESBL) are enzymes produced by some bacteria (Health Protection Agency 2005c). The enzymes are able to destroy

Box 3.10   Questions and answers about MRSA

What is **Staphylococcus aureus** *and what can it do?*

Staphlyococcus aureus is a germ that is harmlessly carried by people on their skin or up their noses without causing an infection. It is carried more easily on skin if that skin is broken or there is a rash, cut or sore. *Staphylococcus aureus* may cause wound infections, abscesses and boils.

What is MRSA and what can it do?

MRSA is a form of *Staphylococcus aureus* that is resistant to a number of antibiotics. Like *Staphylococcus aureus* it can cause infections such as wound infections, abscesses and boils. The infections caused by MRSA are no more serious than a normal *Staphylococcus aureus* but they may be harder to treat.

Do I need to stay away from other people?

The patient may have had a recent episode in hospital or have a relative in hospital who has had MRSA and has been isolated. As a rule, patients in hospital are more vulnerable to infection than are the general public. The practice nurse needs to explain that, although MRSA does not cause many problems in the community, patients in hospital with MRSA are isolated to prevent spread of the infection to other hospital inpatients.

Can I still see my family?

People with MRSA in the community should be encouraged to lead a normal life. There is no reason why relatives and friends who are fit and healthy should stay away from patients with MRSA. If relatives are concerned about their own health, they should be advised to speak to their general practitioner or the local infection control nurse. All relatives should be reminded about basic hygiene precautions such as covering cuts and grazes, and attention to hand washing.

Can it be treated?

MRSA can usually be treated successfully.

How can I stop MRSA spreading?

The main route of transmission is on people's hands so patients should be reminded about the importance of hand washing and should, if necessary, be taught a good technique.

Do I need to take special precautions with my laundry?

Laundry should be washed in the hottest wash the material can stand.

a large number of commonly used antibiotics making the bacteria very resistant and the infections they cause hard to treat. The bacteria associated with ESBL are *Klebsiella* and *Escherichia coli (E. coli)*. Klebsiella ESBL was mainly found in hospitalised patients on specialist areas such as Intensive Therapy Units (ITUs). ESBL producing *E.coli* occurs in both community and hospital patients. The Health Protection Agency recommends that there is good communication between microbiologists and GPs so that local practices are aware if they are in an area of high ESBL prevalence and can therefore take appropriate action with regard to samples and treatment. The practice nurse should promote the importance of hygiene within the patient's home. Prescribers should ensure that antibiotics are only prescribed when needed at the right dose and for the correct duration.

Some of the questions that the practice nurse is likely to be asked are listed in Box 3.11 with appropriate responses

Infestations

Head lice

In recent years the numbers of head lice infections appear to have increased. Whether it is increased awareness and revulsion against lice or a genuine increase is uncertain. Parents who find that they or their children have a head lice infection certainly need reassurance. With correct treatment and aftercare, lice can be kept at bay.

It may sometimes be important to put head lice information into perspective – head lice do not kill; they are a nuisance and no more. The amount of confusion amongst the general population at large and healthcare professionals may also add to the panic about head lice (Olowokure, Jenkinson, Beaumont & Duggal 2003). Practice nurses need to be aware of the facts about lice to enable them to explain clearly to their patients and dispel myths and fears. Readers should familiarise themselves with local policy with regard to head lice, which can be obtained from local Health Protection Units or PCT. New national guidance is awaited, which will update the 1998 guidelines (Aston, Duggal & Simpson 1998).

Facts about lice

Head lice are greyish-brown wingless insects, approximately 2–3 mm long, which live, breed and die on human scalps. They like to stay close to the scalp for warmth, and feed by biting the scalp and sucking the blood. The eggs are grey, the size of a pin head and enclosed in a sac that is 'glued' to the base of the hair near the scalp. After seven days, a young louse (nymph)

Box 3.11   Questions and answers about ESBL

What is E. coli and what can it do?

E. coli is a bacterium that is part of the normal body flora and is found in the bowel. *E. coli* only cause infection if they get into the wrong part of the body. *E. coli* most often cause urinary tract infections (UTIs), but may sometimes progress to blood poisoning that can be life threatening.

What is ESBL producing **E. coli?**

These are antibiotic resistant strains of *E. coli* that have the capability of causing infections in the same way as a normal *E. coli* but they are much harder to treat.

Is the infection caused by ESBL treatable?

In many instances only two oral antibiotics and a very limited group of intravenous antibiotics remain effective.

Are some people more at risk than others?

Most of the infections have occurred in people who are already very sick, elderly, taking antibiotics or have previously been in hospital.

How can I stop it spreading?

Basic hygiene measures will help in stopping it spreading. The risk of acquiring infections is small but it is always good practice to ensure basic hygiene is observed. This includes:

- thorough hand hygiene
- thorough cleansing of cuts and grazes
- regular bathing/showering
- regular changing of linen, including underwear
- family members to use their own flannels, towels, toothbrushes, razors
- safe handling, storage and cooking of food.

will hatch and leave the egg shell (nit), which turns white and grows out with the hair unless physically removed. Head lice are fully mature after 10 days and can live for up to four weeks. The female may lay as many as 10 eggs a day.

Head lice cannot fly and do not jump. They need warmth and do not survive away from the scalp. Transmission occurs through close head-to-head contact where the louse walks from one head to another using its claws to hang on to the strands of hair.

Detection of head lice

Parents of school-age children must be advised to check their children's hair on a regular basis (preferably weekly) during holidays as well as term time. Itching may be a sign of infection, but it may take up to three months for the bites to irritate; therefore parents should be encouraged to look for live lice on the child's head and not wait for itching to start. It is far easier and less painful to inspect hair that is wet and has conditioner applied. Lice are unable to move quickly in wet hair and are therefore easier to find. The procedure for checking hair is summarised in Box 3.12.

Box 3.12   Procedure for checking hair for head lice

- Hair should be parted into sections, and each section should be inspected thoroughly before moving on to the next to ensure that the whole head is inspected.
- Hair should be combed using a plastic detection comb, starting at the root of the hair and combing right to the end.
- Hair should be combed over a white surface such as a sink or piece of white paper.
- Eggs and nits may be observed during combing; they resemble dandruff and cannot be combed out.
- Squeezing the egg between the finger and thumb and drawing it along the hair shaft should remove eggs and nits.
- When all the hair has been combed, the detection comb and the white surface should be inspected for lice.
- Treatment should be commenced as soon as possible only if live head lice are found.
- The index case must be encouraged to inform close contacts so that they can check for head lice and treat if necessary.

Treatment

The three forms of treatment available in 2007 were insecticides, wet combing and a non-insecticidal ointment that coats the head lice and interferes with the water balance in lice (British National Formulary 2007). Advise parents that reinfestation is common, especially when the child is in contact with a peer who has not been treated.

The control of head lice is achieved through a multidisciplinary approach. School health advisers provide education in schools through clinics, leaflets and pre-school meetings with parents. Parents may also approach their health visitor, practice nurse, community pharmacist, general practitioner or local Health Protection Unit for further advice.

Scabies

Scabies has been a common disease for at least 3000 years. It has been associated with being 'dirty' and perhaps promiscuous. The truth, however, is that scabies is caught by prolonged skin-to-skin contact with an infected person and can affect anyone in the population. Outbreaks of infection often occur in residential homes and special schools where residents are at particular risk because of close living and working conditions.

Facts about scabies

Scabies infection is an allergic reaction to the presence of *Sarcoptes scabiei*, which is a mite that burrows into the skin in humans. Scabies infection also occurs in other animals, but the scabies mite is specific to each animal. The egg is laid in the burrow and hatches within 3–5 days. The mature mite lays two or three eggs each day; this can go on for nearly two months. Larvae and nymphs leave the burrow and find protection in hair follicles. The mite burrows into the skin using its legs and mouth parts. The female mite usually spends the rest of her life in the burrow, whereas the immature forms and young adults spend time in the burrows and on the skin surface, from where they can pass to a new host. It is probable that the successful infection of a new host is made possible by the transference of a fertilised female.

The mites can be removed from the burrows by the finger nails during an intensive scratch and can be killed, although sometimes the top of the burrow is scraped away without damage to the mite, which moves out of this position and burrows again.

Transmission

The mite is transferred from one person to another through prolonged skin-to-skin contact. This is most common in families, between healthcare staff and patients, while holding hands and during intimate contact. The two types of scabies infection, caused by the same mite, are classical scabies and crusted Norwegian or hyperkeratotic scabies.

Classical infection

Classical scabies infection is found in healthy people with normal immune systems; the mites are few in number.

A primary infection will normally have no symptoms for up to six weeks following infection. When the patient becomes sensitised to the mite, the symptoms will appear, and an inconspicuous, extremely itchy rash will develop. It is not uncommon for people to scratch themselves until they bleed.

The burrows are usually found between the webs of fingers, around the nipples, occasionally the soles of the feet. The accompanying rash is bilateral and symmetrical and may be found on any or all of the following: wrists and forearms; axillary folds; sides of the thorax; around the waist and the lower quadrants of the buttocks; the insides of legs and ankles. Nodules may develop at sites such as the elbows, anterior axillary folds, penis and scrotum. They are intensely itchy and may continue for weeks or months after successful treatment. Following the primary rash and intense scratching, secondary bacterial infection may occur in the breaks in the skin.

Crusted Norwegian or hyperkeratotic scabies

This form of scabies occurs in people whose immune systems can mount little or no defence against the mite. There are an enormous number of mites present on the host, numbering thousands.

The skin becomes crusty and is often unsightly, but although the patient may feel some discomfort, the rash is not itchy and may appear anywhere on the body if it appears at all. Patients with Norwegian scabies are extremely infectious and can often be the cause of outbreaks of classical scabies amongst close contacts.

Treatment of scabies

Usually an aqueous-based insecticidal lotion is applied to the whole body and left in place for 12–24 hours depending on the product (British National Formulary 2007). A patient who requires treatment should be advised to get someone to help them in order to ensure that the whole body is thoroughly covered in the treatment. Attention should be paid to the hands. Nails should be cut short and treatment applied under them using cotton buds. Care should be taken to ensure that the lotion does not get in to the eyes. Oral therapy is available but only on a named patient basis and can be used in cases where lotions have proved ineffective.

The close contacts of those who are infected also require treatment, even if they are not displaying symptoms, because of the long incubation period. All close contacts should be identified and everyone should be treated on the same day to prevent re-infection. Close contacts are:

- those living under the same roof
- the index case's partner
- in institutions, clients and care staff who have been in contact with the infected person; in some instances this will include all staff in a home.

Reasons for prolonged infection

Treatment failure may occur if the lotion has not been applied thoroughly to all parts of the body. The skin should not be washed during the treatment. If skin, such as hands, needs to be washed, the treatment must be reapplied.

Incomplete contact tracing

It is important that all close contacts are identified and treated at the same time as the infected person, whether or not they are displaying symptoms. This is necessary to prevent reinfection occurring due to the long incubation period.

The role of the practice nurse in the treatment of head lice and scabies

The practice nurse is in an ideal situation to advise patients on contact tracing and how to use treatments effectively. Equally important, the practice nurse can reassure, educate and dispel myths. Literature should be available, and informative posters displayed at peak times might also be helpful. These can be obtained through pharmaceutical companies. (For more information on head lice and scabies see Burgess 1995, 1996.)

Notifiable diseases

The diagnosing doctor should notify the proper officer, usually based in the public health department, of certain diseases (Table 3.6). It is a legal requirement for which the doctor receives a fee. Notification of disease is an important part of the surveillance and monitoring of different diseases, although it is recognised that there is underreporting.

Table 3.6   Statutorily notifiable diseases

Under the Public Health (Control of disease) Act 1984
Cholera
Plague
Relapsing fever
Smallpox
Typhus

Under the Public Health (Infectious Diseases) Regulations 1988
Anthrax
Diphtheria
Dysentery (amoebic or bacillary)
Food poisoning
Leprosy
Leptospirosis
Malaria
Measles
Meningitis
Meningococcal septicaemia (without meningitis)
Mumps
Ophthalmia neonatorum
Paratyphoid
Acute Poliomyelitis
Rabies
Rubella
Scarlet fever
Tetanus
Tuberculosis
Typhoid fever
Viral hepatitis
Whooping cough
Yellow fever

Local consultants in communicable disease control have the powers to add other diseases to the list within their area, but this has to be done through the local law courts. Details of infectivity and the exclusion needs of communicable diseases can be found in the Appendix to this chapter.

Summary

This chapter has briefly summarised areas within general practice where the practice nurse can influence infection control. The infection control guidelines, if followed, will ensure safety of both patients and staff.

It would be unrealistic to expect immediate major changes in practice policy, but nurses must exercise their accountability to themselves, patients, employers and colleagues by identifying areas in which infection control could be improved. No matter how efficient a general practice considers itself, a closer scrutiny may elicit some unwelcome home truths. Self-assessment and audit tools are available within the *Essential Steps to Safe Clean Care* documentation (Department of Health 2006c) and will assist the practice in assessing how well they are doing with the national infection control standards and what remains as outstanding work to do.

All staff must be aware of infection control policies; this requires a good communication channel to ensure that ancillary staff follow the recommended guidelines.

The local PCT and the infection prevention and control nurses and the local Health Protection Unit are the main resources for support, literature and data on local infectious diseases and should be approached for further information.

Key points

- Infection control is the responsibility of all staff.
- Risk assessment of the current practice might identify areas for improvement. Nurses must keep abreast of emerging infections to be informed and support their patients.

Suggested reading

Ayliffe GAJ, Fraise AP, Geddes AM & Mitchell K (2000) *Control of Hospital Infection: A Practical Handbook*, 4th edn. London: Arnold.

Department of Health (2006) *The Health Act: Code of Practice for the Prevention and Control of Healthcare Associated Infections*. London: Department of Health.

Department of Health (2006) *Saving Lives, High Impact intervention No1 2006, Essential Steps to Safe, Clean Care*. London: Department of Health.

Department of Health (2006) *Essential Steps to Safe Clean Care: Reducing Healthcare Associated Infections in Primary Care Trusts, Mental Health Trusts; Learning Disability Organisations; Independent Healthcare; Care Homes' Hospices; GP Practices and Ambulance Services*. London: Department of Health.

Infection Control Nurses Association (2003) *Infection Control Guidance for General Practice*. London: Infection Control Nurses Association.

Useful websites

www.hpa.org.uk
www.dh.gov.uk

Appendix

Table A.1   Periods of exclusion for infectious disease

Disease	Exclusion of patients	Management of home contacts
Chickenpox	Minimum period of exclusion five days from onset of rash	Pregnant women should seek advice from their own doctor
Cold sores (Herpes Simplex Type 1)	None Very young children may spread the virus by touching infected sore	None Towels and face cloths should not be shared
Conjunctivitis	None	None Towels and face cloths should not be shared
Diarrhoea and/or vomiting	All cases to be excluded from school or work until they have been free from diarrhoea for 48 hours	None
E. coli O157	Seek advice from the local Health Protection Unit	Seek advice from the local Health Protection Unit. Stool specimens will be required. Environmental Health Officers will co-ordinate this
German measles (Rubella)	Minimum period of exclusion five days from onset of rash	Pregnant women should seek advice from their own doctor
Hand, foot and mouth	None Children should be well enough to attend school	Close watch to be kept on contacts. It can be transmitted to nearby persons by direct contact, droplet spread and faecal orally. Basic hygiene must be observed
Hepatitis A (Jaundice)	Seek advice from the local Health Protection Unit Exclusion may be necessary in some cases	None, but any contacts showing signs of being unwell should seek medical advice
Hepatitis B and C	None Case may attend when well enough. Not infectious under normal school/work conditions	Household contacts of cases of Hepatitis B may require follow up and vaccinating
HIV infection	None Case may attend if well enough. Not infectious under normal school/work conditions	

Table A.1 *Continued*

Disease	Exclusion of patients	Management of home contacts
Impetigo	Exclude until lesions are crusted or healed. This process may be speeded up by antibiotics	None
Measles	Minimum period of exclusion five days from onset of rash	None
Acute meningitis and septicaemia	Until considered by General Medical Practitioner to be free from infection and <u>fit</u> to return to school/work	Household contacts may be offered antibiotics. Close contacts of meningitis do not need to be excluded from school / nursery, etc
Molluscum contagiosum	None, but avoid contact with the lesions	None
MRSA	None unless patient is unwell	Household contacts should be reminded about good hygiene including hand washing and environmental cleaning to minimise spread
Mumps	Minimum period of exclusion until swelling has subsided (five days minimum)	None
Parvoviruses infection (Fifth Disease or Slapped Cheek Syndrome)	None	Women who may be pregnant should seek advice from their own doctor
Pediculosis (Infection of hair with lice)	None	Follow up of household and close contacts is essential
Ringworm of the body and head	Exclusion not normally necessary during treatment unless specifically advised by the Health Protection Unit	Enquire about household and close contacts. Check and treat symptomatic pets
Ringworm of feet (athlete's foot)	Exclusion from barefoot activities unnecessary but treatment always advisable	None
Scabies	Cases can return to school or work after first treatment	Careful follow up and contact tracing are essential especially close family and social contacts. Contacts require treatment
Shingles	Exclude only if rash is weeping and cannot be covered	Non-immune people can catch chickenpox from patients with shingles as it is the same virus

Table A.1   *Continued*

Disease	Exclusion of patients	Management of home contacts
Streptococcal infection (Scarlet Fever)	Until clinically recovered and pronounced fit by General Medical Practitioner, or five days after commencing antibiotic therapy if well enough to return	None
Threadworm	None	Treat all family contacts. Strict attention to hand hygiene in school and home
Tuberculosis (primary and secondary)	At the discretion of the chest physician. Normally excluded from school/work and not allowed to return until declared to be noninfectious by a chest physician	Contacts showing no signs of tuberculosis need not be excluded, as they will in any case be under medical supervision
Typhoid fever and paratyphoid fever	Exclusion is important for some people in certain risk groups. Advice is available from the local Health Protection Unit	The Head Teacher will be informed regarding freedom from infection and re-admission of siblings and other contacts who work at school including food handlers
Verrucae (plantar warts)	Exclusion is not necessary provided the warts remain covered with occlusive plaster. People with plantar warts need not be excluded from swimming and other barefoot activities provided the warts remain covered with occlusive plaster	None
Whooping cough (Pertussis)	Minimum period of exclusion 21 days from onset of paroxysmal cough. Reduced to five days if given antibiotics	None

Adapted from Health Protection Agency 2006

References

Adu FD, Adedeji AA, Essan JS & Odusanya OG (1996) Live viral vaccine potency: an index for assessing the cold chain system. *Public Health* 110, 325–330.

Aston R, Duggal H & Simpson J 'The Stafford Group' (1998) *Guidance on Managing Head Lice Infection in Children*. Public Health Medicine and Environmental Group. www.phmeg.org.uk/documents/headlice (accessed June 2007).

Ayliffe GAJ, Lowbury EJL, Geddes AM & Williams JD (Eds) (1992) *Control of Hospital Infection: A Practical Handbook*. London: Chapman and Hall.

Bowell B (1992) A risk to others. *Nursing Times* 88(4), 38–40.

British National Formulary (2007) *BNF No 53*. London: Royal Pharmaceutical Society of Great Britain/BMJ Publishing Group.

Burgess IF (1995) Human lice and their management. *Advances in Parasitology* 36, 271–342.

Burgess IF (1996) Management guidelines for lice and scabies. *Prescriber* 7(90), 87–99.

Chief Medical Officer (2007) *Changes to the mandatory healthcare associated infection surveillance system for Clostridium difficile associated diarrhoea from April 2007*. London: Department of Health.

Department of Health (2004) *HIV Post-exposure Prophylaxis: Guidance from the UK Chief Medical Officers Expert Advisory Group on AIDS*. www.dh.gov.uk (accessed June 2007).

Department of Health (2006a) *The Health Act: Code of Practice for the Prevention and Control of Healthcare Associated Infections*. London: Department of Health.

Department of Health (2006b) *Saving Lives, High Impact Intervention No1 2006, Essential Steps to Safe, Clean Care*. London: Department of Health.

Department of Health (2006c) *Essential Steps to Safe Clean Care: Reducing Healthcare Associated Infections in Primary Care Trusts, Mental Health Trusts; Learning Disability Organisations; Independent Healthcare; Care Homes' Hospices; GP Practices and Ambulance Services*. London: Department of Health.

Department of Health (2006d) *Environment and Sustainability. Health Technical Memorandum 07-01 Safe Management of Healthcare Waste*. London: The Stationery Office.

Department of Health (2006e) *Immunisation Against Infectious Diseases, 3rd edn*. London: The Stationary Office.

Foy C, Gallagher M & Rhodes T (1990) HIV and measures to control infection in general practice. *Journal of Hospital Infection* 3, 29–37.

Gould D (1995) Infection control: survey to determine nurses' knowledge in a clinical setting. *Nursing Standard* 9(36), 35–38.

Healthcare Commission (2006) *Investigation into outbreaks of* Clostridium difficile *at Stoke Mandeville Hospital, Buckinghamshire Hospitals NHS Trust*. London: Commission for Healthcare Audit and Inspection.

Health Protection Agency (2005a) *The Eye of the Needle: Surveillance of Significant Occupational Exposure to Blood Borne Viruses in Healthcare Workers. Centre for Infections; England, Wales and Northern Ireland Seven Year Report*. London: Health Protection Agency.

Health Protection Agency (2005b) *Results of the Voluntary Reporting Scheme for* Clostridium difficile *in England, Wales and Northern Ireland 1995–2004: Trend in Total Reports*. www.hpa.org.uk /topics (accessed 12 September 2007).

Health Protection Agency (2005c) *Investigations into Multi-drug Resistant ESBL Producing* Escherichia coli *Strains Causing Infection in England*. www.hpa.org.uk/ publications (accessed June 2006).

Health Protection Agency (2006) *Guidance on Infection Control in Schools and Other Child Care Settings*. London: Prolog.

Health Protection Agency PVL Working Group (2006) *Interim Guidance on Diagnosis and Management of PVL-associated Staphylococcal Infections in the UK. London:* Department of Health. www.dh.gov.uk (accessed June 2007).

Health and Safety Executive (1994) *Control of Substances Hazardous to Health Regulations (Revised)*. London: HMSO.

Hoffman PN, Cooke EM & Larkin DP (1988) Control of infection on general practice: a survey and recommendations. *British Medical Journal* 297, 34–36.

Infection Control Nurses Association (2003) *Infection Control Guidance for General Practice*. London: ICNA.

National Audit Office (2000) *The Management and Control of Hospital Acquired Infection in NHS Acute Trusts in England: Report by the Comptroller and Auditor General – HC 230 Session 1999–2000*. London: The Stationery Office.

National Clostridium difficile Standards Group (2003) Report to the Department of Health. *Journal of Hospital Infection* 56 Suppl 1, 1–38.

National Health Service Confederation/BMA (2003) *New GMS Contract. Investing in General Practice*. London: NHS Confederation/BMA.

National Patient Safety Agency (2006) *National Colour Coding Scheme for Hospital Cleaning Materials and Equipment*. London: NHS.

Nightingale F (1859) *Notes on Nursing: What it is and What it is not*. London: Harrison.

Office of National Statistics (2006) Report: Deaths involving *Clostridium difficile:* England and Wales, 1999–2004. *Health Statistics Quarterly* 30, Spring.

Olowokure B, Jenkinson H, Beaumont M & Duggal H (2003) The knowledge of healthcare professionals with regard to the treatment and prevention of head lice. *International Journal of Environmental Health Research* 13 (1), 11–15.

Pratt RJ, Pellowe CM, Wilson JA, Loveday HP, Harper PJ, Jones SRLJ, McDougall C & Wilcox MH (2007) epic2: National evidence-based guidelines for preventing healthcare-associated infections in NHS hospitals in England. *Journal of Hospital Infection* 655, s1–s64.

Royal College of Nursing (2005) *Good Practice in Infection Prevention and Control: Guidance for Nursing Staff*. London: RCN.

Taylor LJ (1978) An evaluation of hand washing techniques, Part 2 *Nursing Times* 74 (1), 108–110.

UK Health Departments (1990) *Guidance for Clinical Healthcare Workers: Protection against infection with HIV and Hepatitis Viruses. Recommendations of the Expert Advisory group on AIDS*. London: HMSO.

Chapter 4

Health Promotion

Diana Forster, Diane Pannell and Marilyn Edwards

Health promotion plays a major role in helping to maximise the future health of the nation. It should be undertaken following an assessment of the needs of a practice population to ensure strategies are planned appropriately and resources are targeted effectively. The first part of this chapter explains how to assess needs; the process has not changed since the first edition. The latter part of the chapter places health promotion into context within two specific health agendas.

The pre-conception health of both mother and father will influence fertility, the viability of a conception and the outcome of the pregnancy. It is hoped that the issues discussed within this chapter will increase practice nurse awareness and subsequent pre-conception health advice.

Finally, we shall consider osteoporosis, which is a major cause of fractures in the elderly, having cost implications for the individual, health and social services. Targeted health promotion can help both in delaying the onset of the disease, and in improving compliance in management when the disease is established.

Theories and models of health promotion can be found in excellent health promotion textbooks and are therefore not discussed in this chapter.

Needs assessment

The assessment of health needs has a vital part to play in the current climate of a primary care-led National Health Service. One of the key roles of health authorities is to understand how healthy their relevant population is, and what its health needs are. Limited available resources should be allocated on a basis of need, although most healthcare is now Government-led.

The provision of healthcare by interdisciplinary, primary healthcare teams is expanding in scope and importance, rather than being seen merely

The Informed Practice Nurse, Edwards, M. (2008), Chichester: Wiley.

as a gatekeeper to secondary care. The practice nurse has a key role in assessing the healthcare needs of the practice population that must then be shared with the wider practice team and Primary Care Trust if appropriate.

A public health approach

Health professionals increasingly work from both a public health and a personal healthcare perspective. This means assessing needs and trends in the health and disease patterns of populations as distinct from individuals. Health is increasingly viewed as a personal, family and community responsibility.

Epidemiological data from a variety of sources provides a picture of healthcare needs. Demographers collate data about people who live in a geographical area, including their age and gender, and annual birth, death, marriage and morbidity figures. Box 4.1 provides definitions of epidemiology and demography.

In order to build a picture of health needs, service users should be included when planning, publishing information and monitoring performance. Patients can verbalise local need through Patient Advocacy Liaison Service (PALS), and at Primary Care Trust public meetings. Primary care-led local services should be aware of health needs from a public health perspective, not just reacting to patient demands, but also considering the wider population's needs. For primary healthcare workers overwhelmed by patient demand, this can be difficult, as illustrated in the Activity 4.1. These dilemmas are still relevant in 2008.

Box 4.1   Epidemiology and demography (Farmer, Miller & Lawrenson 1996)

Epidemiology: from the Greek, literally meaning 'studies upon people'. The principle uses of epidemiology have been summarised as:

- the investigation of the causes and natural history of disease, with the aim of disease prevention and health promotion
- the measurement of healthcare needs and the evaluation of clinical management, with the aim of improving the effectiveness and efficiency of healthcare provision.

Demography: the study of whole populations of people.

Activity 4.1

Consider the following dilemmas (Harris 1996):
Should a chronically neurotic woman with a marital problem occupy as much of her GP's time as it would take the GP to do annual domiciliary diabetic checks on non-attendees at the practice?
Should attendees in a practice be screened opportunistically for diabetes, while the majority of the elderly population who may suffer disability from hearing loss are not screened for this, going without adequate hearing assessment or provision of aids and education?

Client's views

Although incorporating user's views of need into the planning of services has received increasing attention, there are methodological difficulties in obtaining service user's views and including them in the policy process. Ethical issues are raised when needs are uncovered which cannot be met in practice because of resource constraints (Billings & Cowley 1995).

Difficult choices and policy decisions have to be made when needs are inexhaustible while resources are not. Some examples were presented in the dilemmas above. Similarly, practice nurses often use their knowledge and influence to address the complex needs of homeless people. A report about tuberculosis and homeless people (Griffiths-Jones 1997) highlighted the following comprehensive needs:

- reducing the number of homeless people and improving available accommodation
- improving nutrition through health education and support
- the early identification of tuberculosis in homeless people and prompt, successful treatment
- a thorough contact tracing programme.

The main benefits for homeless clients occur when they receive appropriate assessments from practice and community nurses that identify health and social needs followed up by effective referrals. These problems are still pertinent in 2008.

Defining health

Health is notoriously difficult to define. It may be defined negatively as the absence of disease, or in a more positive way as a resource for living. The

WHO's positive definition embraces a holistic approach (WHO 1978). This includes the physical, psychological, emotional and social well-being of a person, group or community.

Health needs therefore encompass education, social services, housing, aspects of the environment and social policy. When estimating health needs it is important to understand what people themselves mean by health.

One study found that health problems were often played down (Bernard & Meade 1993). Typically, older women being interviewed would say 'Oh I'm fine in myself, it's just this . . . stiff knee/high blood pressure/trouble with my waterworks . . . ' Health was being assessed by these women not just in terms of the presence or absence of disease, or in terms of functional ability; the women felt well in spite of their illness or disability.

Blaxter (1990) also found in her research that health could coexist with quite severe disease or incapacity. One woman aged 79 and disabled by arthritis said 'To be well in health means I feel I can do others a good turn if they need help'.

Holistic health

Nurses applying a holistic approach to healthcare place emphasis on the whole person, taking into account physical, emotional, intellectual, spiritual and socio-cultural background.

The concept of need in all these aspects of personal care is highly relevant to nursing. When identifying health needs, the focus is on health promotion, prevention and well-being, helping people to take responsibility for recognising and meeting their own health needs if possible, and influencing local services and policies.

Partnerships between mental health services and local community resources are necessary to meet the increase in people's mental health needs. The need for physical health promotion should not be forgotten for minority groups, such as people with a learning disability or mental health problem.

Defining 'need'

Need is a word frequently used in ordinary conversation. In the context of this chapter, however, need becomes a technical term used in a public health framework. Four main types of need in this sense may be identified, based on Bradshaw's (1972) classification:

Normative needs: are determined or defined by experts or professionals; for example, the components of a healthy diet being explained based on expert research into dietetics, or smoking cessation advice.

Felt needs: are identified by patients, users or carers who want certain services or treatment to be provided, for example, chiropody services.

Expressed needs: are needs translated into action, for instance by someone visiting a clinic or surgery to seek advice or treatment, such as management of a traumatic wound.

Comparative needs: makes comparisons between groups, individuals or areas. This is highlighted in the media with postcode lottery in health-care provision, especially where high cost drugs and treatments are involved.

Whichever type of need is being considered, it is important that accurate and relevant information is available, as a basis for needs assessment at a local or national level. Needs-driven decisions can prevent minority and so-called Cinderella needs being overlooked in favour of patient and professional demands in other areas.

Activity 4.2

Identify the main Cinderella service needs in the vicinity of your home or workplace. Are there ethnic minority groups whose needs for advocacy are not being met, or is there a lack of respite care for carers of both physically and mentally ill people?

Assessing needs for health education

The key to the success of any health teaching activity is identifying the need for it. The nurse may identify a need for diabetic patients to learn how to prevent complications by maintaining as near normal blood glucose levels as possible. Teaching patients to balance their diet with insulin or tablets and making adjustments for the effects of exercise, stress or illness would require the nurse to be an educator, motivator and supporter in meeting such a need.

Similarly, practice nurses may be involved in setting up advisory sessions for potential travellers, when health risks abroad, safety in the sun and required vaccination schedules may be discussed, with the ultimate aim of maintaining current health and preventing future ill health. Ethical issues relating to informed consent for opportunistic health education was raised by Naidoo and Wills (2000 p.127), and should always be considered.

Decision maker or victim?

People have more choice and control over some factors affecting their health needs than others. For example, people can choose whether or not to smoke, but cannot easily control the atmospheric pollution levels to which they are exposed. This includes occupational exposure to any noxious or potentially harmful substance.

Healthcare workers have to understand the personal, community and global web of possible influences on someone's health and well-being in order to assess needs and how to attempt to meet them. For example, smoking is a support mechanism for some people, while a poor diet may be related to inadequate income or management skills.

WHO and primary healthcare

Partnerships with clients, patients and the local community form part of the ongoing movement from secondary to primary healthcare. Since 'Alma Ata' (World Health Organisation 1978), the World Health Organisation has worked for a shift away from medically dominated, acute-focused services. The key to delivering 'Health for all by the year 2000' (World Health Organisation 1978) was identified as primary healthcare, linked to improving basic living conditions (Box 4.2).

The *NHS and Community Care Act* (Department of Health 1990) and the development of NHS Trusts emphasised the change from service-led to

---

Box 4.2   Key principles in the Declaration of Alma-Ata that are vital for assessing and meeting health needs (WHO 1978):

- Accessibility: healthcare that is provided close to where people live and work.
- Acceptability: healthcare that is appropriate and provided in ways that people find acceptable.
- Equity: all people have an equal right to health and healthcare.
- Self-determination: people have the right and the responsibility to make their own health choices.
- Community involvement: people have the right and the responsibility to participate individually and collectively in the planning and implementation of their healthcare.
- A focus on health: primary healthcare concentrates on the promotion of health as well as on the care of people who are sick, frail or disabled.
- A multi-sectoral approach: housing, food policies, environmental policies and social services have an important part to play.

---

needs-led assessment. Purchasers and commissioners became responsible for contracting services appropriate to their local population's needs. Nurses were therefore required to identify specific needs of patients and patient groups.

Primary Care Groups (PCGs) and subsequently Primary Care Trusts (PCTs) were developed to integrate services around the needs of the patients in each locality, tackling the causes of ill health as well as illness and disability. In 2006, PCTs merged to form even larger Trusts, one of whose aims is to engage with its local population to improve its health and well-being (Department of Health 2006a). Practice based commissioning (PBC) was conceived to allow practices to commission services, offering greater freedom and flexibility to tailor services to the needs of the local community (Department of Health 2006b), but has been slow to develop in practice (see Chapter 9).

This approach requires a variety of changes in the ways healthcare is shared out and delivered. It depends on inter-agency working, health promotion, partnerships with patients and clients and above all, on the assessment of health needs.

Practice nurses have a unique part to play in such assessment and are front-line workers in assessing the health needs of people as individuals and as part of a population group.

The 'Health of the Nation Strategy'

The *Health of the Nation* (Department of Health 1992) was an ambitious plan arising out of the theme of 'Health for all by the year 2000' (World Health Organisation 1978). Determining priorities and setting targets were based on an epidemiological assessment of health needs. Since then, the scope has broadened and regular government enquiries investigate current health needs in the UK.

Initial targets were an attempt to meet health needs relating to coronary heart disease and stroke, cancers, mental illness, HIV/AIDS and sexual health and accidents. National Service Frameworks (NSFs) were first launched in 1998 as long-term strategies for improving specific areas of health; they were designed to improve patient care and reduce inequity in service provision (Department of Health 2006c).

Social class and health needs

One of the founding principles of the NHS was that of equal access to healthcare according to need for all citizens, regardless of their position in society or where they lived. However, not all social groups have equal access to healthcare.

Tudor Hart (1971) coined the phrase 'the inverse care law' meaning that health services were generally least available where they were most needed. The greater uptake of preventive and screening services by the non-manual occupations is well documented. Those who actively seek health promotion to meet their health needs are usually those who need it least.

The widening gap in health inequalities

There are many aspects to equality (Figure 4.1). The *Variations in Health* report (Department of Health 1995) pointed out that although mortality rates had fallen steadily, and life expectancy had considerably increased throughout the developed world, there were significant variations in levels of sickness and death between social groups in terms of occupational class, sex, religion and ethnicity, including deaths from preventable diseases. Health inequalities were made a key priority for the NHS in the *Priorities and Planning Framework for 2003–2006* (Department of Health 2006d). The health inequalities targets included life expectancy and infant mortality, with the aim to narrow the health gap in childhood and throughout life between socio-economic groups and between the most deprived areas of the country.

This requires identification of local health inequalities, including improving data quality to identify groups or areas with high health needs or poor

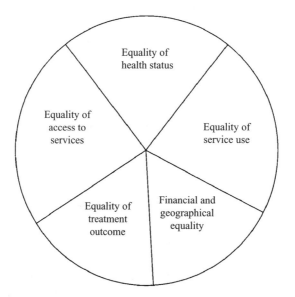

Figure 4.1 Aspects of equality.

health outcomes. Included in the infant mortality is a reduction in teenage pregnancies, improved nutrition in women of childbearing age and a reduction in smoking in pregnancy. The relevance of this is discussed later in the chapter.

Deaths were reported to be least common for babies whose fathers were in the two highest social classes and were more frequent among babies whose fathers were in the lowest (Office for National Statistics 1997). Poor people have less money to spend on nutritious food, clean water, adequate clothing and shelter, which are all essential to a minimum level of health and well-being.

Life expectancy targets include reducing excess winter deaths by promoting influenza vaccination and increasing smoking cessation.

Practice and community profiles

Nurses have a valuable part to play in profiling GP practices to assess health and social needs within the practice population. Teamwork is an essential prerequisite for effective health needs assessment. The individual, family, practice and community health profiles kept by health visitors, and increasingly by other community nurses, form a comprehensive database of people's health experience of healthcare and health needs. The basic principles of health profiling are summarised in Box 4.3.

The information collected within a health profile will vary depending on local circumstances and the type of information. However, most should contain information on:

- Population data – age/sex/ethnicity
- Incidence of disease, illness, disability and trauma and causes of death, for example types of cancer or coronary heart disease
- Information on health service provision, such as take up of immunisation and breast screening
- Social and environmental data such as housing, employment status and number of teenage mothers.

Box 4.3   Four basic principles of health profiling

1. Collecting and analysing information
2. Selecting priorities for action
3. Choosing nursing activities, including methods of working, for selected priorities
4. Evaluating nursing practice.

Box 4.4   Issues to be considered when compiling a community profile (Billingham 1994)

- Monitoring and describing the population's health
- Identifying those groups most in need of health support, guidance and treatment
- Identifying the social, economic and environmental factors that have an impact on people's health
- Taking health action to promote and protect the population's health
- Assessing the impact of healthcare on health.

The five main issues to be considered when compiling a community profile can be seen in Box 4.4.

Gathering data

The age-sex register is one of the most basic pieces of information that is available in every practice. For a comprehensive health needs assessment a wider population than the practice list should be analysed, for instance, comparing national census information or public health reports. Access to computerised health data facilitates the data collection related to chronic diseases such as diabetes, cancers and cardiovascular disease.

The Office for National Statistics (ONS)

The ONS aims to bring together all the important data about the lives of everyone in Britain in a way that makes the information accessible, organising the national system of registering births, deaths and marriages that began in 1837. National, regional and local annual health and population tables are published on separate topics including family statistics, morbidity, population estimates and projections and longitudinal studies. The ONS has the responsibility for the census, which is a major study providing current information that can help to identify health needs and aid future planning.

Census data

Since 1801 there has been a full census every 10 years in Britain, except in 1941 during the Second World War. The collated data shows the changing patterns of populations. All the information can be broken down into smaller statistical tables including health authorities, wards or parishes, and is therefore useful in planning healthcare services and anticipating needs.

Accessing information

Local libraries and the PCT Public Health Departments can be valuable sources of expertise and information, providing publications such as *Social Trends, Population Trends, On the State of the Public Health* and the local Director of Public Health's annual report. The *Public Health Common Data Set* is circulated annually to health authorities by the Institute of Public Health. It contains essential information for identifying people at risk and assessing community health needs. Much of this information can be viewed and downloaded via the Office for National Statistics website.

Integrated nursing

Responding to the full range of population health needs is easier to achieve where integrated nursing teams have been developed. The skills, knowledge and experience of a team that includes practice nurses, district nurses, school nurses, community midwives, mental health nurses and health visitors should enable a wide range of health needs to be identified and prioritised. For example, practice based, multidisciplinary cancer and palliative care meetings are an ideal forum to identify, share and find solutions for individual patient and family needs. Each professional will have a different piece of the puzzle to contribute. Similarly, liaison with midwives and health visitors will benefit prospective mothers.

Promoting pre-conception care

Pre-conception care

Pre-conception care empowers people within the childbearing range to take responsibility for both their own and their future offspring's health. Preventative care may reduce or eliminate some of the more frequent problems relating to unhealthy lifestyle, poor nutrition, substance abuse, or failure to comply with medical treatment, which may have adverse effects on the conception, pregnancy or perinatal morbidity and mortality rates. This was included in the health inequalities targets discussed in the previous section.

Pre-conception screening and interventions are as important as the pregnancy itself in achieving the optimum maternal-fetal outcome (Leuzzi &

Scoles 1996). Ideally the prospective parents would seek advice from health professionals when they plan a pregnancy. However, this is not always the case for those who actively plan a pregnancy and not an issue for those who become unintentionally pregnant.

Men also benefit by reassessing their lifestyle and should be included in pre-conception counselling, as their health will affect the quality of their sperm and fertility. Pre-conceptual care by the professional should be seen as a time to educate, screen, diagnose and treat before pregnancy.

Opportunities for pre-conception health education

The most effective results in preconception care are seen from a planned package of care with the client. There are many areas where the lifestyle of either or both prospective parents affects the fetal well-being (Figure 4.2), and many opportunities for the nurse to promote pre-conception care, for example, at:

- well women / well men clinics
- family planning clinics
- immunisation clinics
- travel vaccination sessions
- pregnancy test results discussions
- new patient health checks
- haematological investigations.

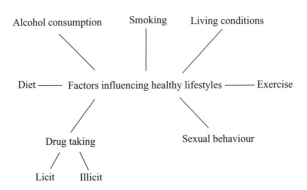

Figure 4.2 Lifestyle factors affecting fetal well-being.

Nutrition and maternal weight

The old adage of we are what we eat, has a greater importance for the pre-conceptual woman. What she eats not only affects her health, but also may directly influence her ability to conceive or carry a pregnancy to term (Figure 4.3).

Women are advised to be within the normal body mass index (BMI) of 20–25 before commencing pregnancy, and are recommended to follow a healthy, well-balanced diet (Buttriss, Wynne & Stanner 2001). A low BMI has been associated with reduced ability to conceive, and the subsequent pregnancy being at risk. Mothers may deliver low birth weight babies who have associated problems, have an increased risk of sudden infant death syndrome, or babies who suffer from respiratory difficulties.

An increased BMI may be due to a medical problem such as polycystic ovary syndrome (PCOS), where ovulation is affected and the ability to conceive reduced. Women with diagnosed PCOS should be referred to their GP for hormonal management and may need referral for specialist advice (Edwards 2006). Conversely, women with PCOS may think themselves unable to conceive, and have an unplanned pregnancy.

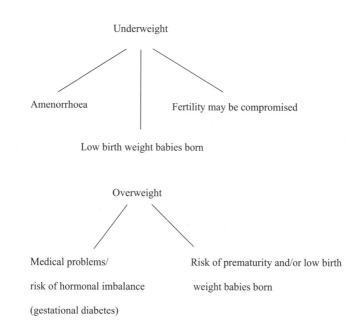

Figure 4.3 Weight and its effects on fertility and fetal well-being.

A woman should be encouraged to attain a normal BMI before conception, with obesity a recognised risk factor for gestational diabetes (Diabetes UK 2006). Dieting during pregnancy may result in nutritional imbalance for the mother and fetus, so weight loss is recommended prior to conception. Exercise is an integral part of weight management and should be encouraged.

What a woman can and cannot eat during a pregnancy is often perceived as a minefield and consequently ignored. If appropriate information is provided beforehand, the parents become more familiar with potentially hazardous foods. While some foods should be avoided, intake of others should be increased.

A raised intake of Vitamin A (retinoids) has been shown to be teratogenic (Department of Health and Social Security 1990), and foods with high levels of this vitamin, such as liver and its by-products, and multivitamin tablets with added vitamin A are to be avoided. Low levels of zinc have been associated with heart defects and growth retardation. Folic acid, however, has been shown to have beneficial effects on the fetus, reducing the incidence of neural tube defects (see below).

The identification and rebalance of nutritional inadequacies preconceptionally will provide a healthier outcome for mother and baby.

Folic acid

Folates and folic acid have been conclusively identified as reducing the risk of neural tube defects, such as spina bifida and anencephaly, in developing babies (Medical Research Council Vitamin Study Group 1991). The neural tube (brain and spine) is developed within the first 23–26 days after conception, generally before the woman is aware of a pregnancy. Women are advised to take a 400 mcg daily folic acid supplement, and increase their intake of dietary folates, giving a total of 600 mcg of folic acid/folate, for at least three months before conception and for the first 12 weeks of pregnancy (British Nutrition Foundation 2002; Department of Health 2000, 2006e).

Women who have had a baby with a neural tube abnormality are advised to take 5 mgs of folic acid daily and increase their dietary folates (Box 4.5) (Prodigy 2006a). Leaflets and dietary fact-sheets to supplement verbal advice should be made readily available in surgery waiting-areas. Information can also be downloaded from the Department of Health and British Nutrition Foundation websites.

In the United States of America it has been suggested that folic acid be added to oral contraceptives in an attempt to reach the many women who have unplanned pregnancies, as remembering to take an additional pill every day is a barrier expressed by women in folic acid campaign focus groups (Verbiest 2005). Watch the nursing and medical press to see if this

---

Box 4.5   Examples of foods containing folates (Buttriss et al. 2001)

Vegetables: broccoli, brussel sprouts, cabbage, cauliflower, green beans, peas, potatoes, spinach, sweetcorn, lettuce, tomatoes

Most fruits: bananas, grapefruit, oranges, orange juice

Cereals: brown rice, spaghetti, bread, breakfast cereals fortified with folic acid

Other foods: marmite, Bovril, yeast extract, milk (whole or semi-skimmed), yoghurt some breakfast cereals and bread have added folic acid

---

becomes practice – what happens in the USA is usually replicated in the UK at a later date. It is likely that folic acid will be added to bread flour in 2007 in another attempt to protect the unborn child (British Nutrition Foundation 2006).

Environmental and lifestyle hazards

Areas that have a great influence on health, and which can be addressed pre-conceptionally include smoking, alcohol, drugs and infections.

Smoking

Smoking and its associated health problems are well documented. Less publicised is the knowledge that smoking can cause an increased risk of infertility. Male fertility is compromised as sperm from smokers has been found to be decreased in density and motility compared with nonsmokers (Wynn & Wynn 1991). Impotence is not uncommon in smokers, due to vascular changes reducing the blood flow necessary for an erection. Men may be more inclined to stop smoking if aware of these vascular changes.

Women who smoke are at risk not only of delayed conception but also an increased risk of early miscarriage, low birth weight baby, placental abruption, lifelong disabilities and sudden infant death syndrome (Economides & Braithwaite 1994; Moos 2004; Schoendorf & Kiely 1992).

Alcohol

Alcohol has been shown to adversely affect sperm and ova by affecting the rate of conception and its viability (Crawley 1993). One single episode of alcohol abuse around the time of conception has been shown to affect fetal brain growth, and increases the risk of congenital malformations.

Women who drink more than six units a day are at risk of their baby developing fetal alcohol syndrome, which is characterised by physical abnormalities and intellectual impairment (Ernhart et al. 1987; Rolater, Winslow & Jaconson 2000). Heavy drinkers who decrease their alcohol intake preconceptionally can reduce the risk of intrauterine growth retardation, but not congenital malformations (Day, Jasperse & Richardson 1989). In these instances, it is essential to work together with the potential parents, and agencies such as Alcoholics Anonymous to afford the best healthcare for the parent and baby. The advice to avoid alcohol altogether as no safe limits have been given (Rolater et al. 2000), or minimise drinking to 1–2 units once or twice a week (Prodigy 2006a), is reinforced by the Department of Health (2007), but as this discrepancy is confusing, it would be advisable for the woman to consume minimal alcohol intake pre-conception and none during the pregnancy.

Drugs

Commercially prepared and illegal drugs can affect the developing fetus, particularly during organ development. Consequently women are advised to avoid intake of any drug. Women who require medication for medical conditions should seek advice from their doctor. Diabetics require specialist advice. It is essential to remember that herbal medications and over-the-counter medicines can be harmful in pregnancy (Prodigy 2006a), so raise the topic when discussing medications, and refer the woman to the GP or midwife for advice if necessary.

Illicit drugs are harmful to the mother and the fetus, although the extent largely depends on the drugs taken, and at what gestation. Heroin use affects menstruation and ovulation by disrupting the menstrual cycle, though this returns to normal when heroin is stopped or replaced with methadone, but does not prevent pregnancy (Henderson 1995). Babies born to opiate users tend to be of lower birth weight, and there is increased incidence of antepartum haemorrhage and intrauterine death, which may result from the opiates or the woman's reduced nutritional state (Keen & Alison 2001). Pre-conception counselling for drug misusers should focus on stopping or reducing the illicit drug(s), and improving nutrition to maximise the mother's health. If not already in a drug programme, referral to a drugs agency may be appropriate.

Anabolic steroid use has been linked with sperm damage, though the effects decrease when the drug is stopped. Men should be aware that taken drugs may be secreted in their semen and thus may greatly affect fetal development (Vallance 1996). It may be relevant to discuss this aspect of drug use

Table 4.1 Effects of toxoplasmosis on pregnancy

Time	Effect
First 3 months	risk of miscarriage
3rd–6th months	risk of hydrocephalus and brain lesions causing severe mental retardation and epilepsy
Effects which may not become evident until the child is older	retinochorditis, which may cause partial sightedness or blindness

with the male partner, especially if he uses the gym or is a body builder (Edwards 2006).

Infections

Some infections, while not causing fertility problems, need to be addressed pre-conceptionally. The consequences of some infections can have disastrous effects on the both the pregnancy and fetal well-being.

Toxoplasmosis

Although strictly speaking toxoplasmosis cannot cause infertility, it can adversely affect pregnancy (Table 4.1). *Toxoplasmosis gondii* is a microscopic parasitic infection spread predominately through domestic cat faeces, and from eating undercooked meats.

The symptoms are similar to flu, so a healthy person may be unaware that they have been infected. The parasite can lay dormant in a human causing no further problems until reactivated if the immune system is stressed; for example, during pregnancy. A woman with a first infection of toxoplasmosis is advised to avoid pregnancy for six months.

Congenital toxoplasmosis results from an acute infection acquired by the mother during pregnancy (Centers for Disease Control and Prevention 2006). A small percentage of infected newborns have serious eye or brain damage at birth. General advice is to take special care when handling cats and litter trays, wear gloves when gardening, and wash hands after handling raw meat. All meats should be thoroughly cooked. Further information on the consequences of toxoplasmosis can be obtained from the website listed at the end of the chapter.

Rubella

Rubella is generally thought of as a childhood infection, although any age group can be at risk. Although rubella does not prevent conception,

Table 4.2   Fetal abnormalities due to rubella infection

Stage of gestation	Effect
3–7 weeks gestation	eye lens develops; cataracts are a typical sign of infection microphthalmos (uncommon) pigmentary retinopathy: common but does not affect the sight
6–8weeks	heart; structural abnormalities
2–4 months	ear: hearing problems common in congenital rubella

Low birth weight babies – due to the placenta being inefficient
Transient damage – changes in the bones, especially the long bones; pupera, often accompanied by enlarged liver/spleen; jaundice and inflamed lungs are fairly common side effects

problems arise if a woman becomes infected prior to a pregnancy being confirmed. A fetus under 12 weeks gestation exposed to maternal rubella is at most risk of developing abnormalities, as the infection may interfere with organ development.

The rubella vaccination programme for girls was stopped in 1996, and replaced with two doses of measles, mumps and rubella (MMR) vaccine. The vaccination programme in the UK ensures that most women, and many younger men, have been vaccinated against rubella infections. Vaccine-induced antibodies can persist for 18 years, after which the level of immunity may not be adequate to protect a developing fetus from infection. Many women are delaying having children until their late 20s and 30s and may have lost their immunity, or may not have been immunised (Edwards 2006).

When planning a baby, women should be offered a blood test to check they are rubella immune. If the result is negative, immunisation with MMR is recommended, after which the woman should be advised not to get pregnant for one month (Department of Health 2006f). Vaccine-induced rubella cannot be transmitted to other people but may affect a fetus. A maternal infection does not always mean the fetus will be affected, and abnormalities will depend on the gestation of the infection (Table 4.2).

Vaginal infections

It may be appropriate to offer a woman testing for vaginal infections before conception, even if she is in a stable relationship. This requires sensitive counselling to advise that some infections are asymptomatic and may have been present for some years. Any woman at risk of sexually transmitted infections (STIs) should be referred to a genito-urinary medicine (GUM) clinic for diagnosis, management and contact tracing. Referrals may be via the practice nurse, GP or self-referral. High vaginal swabs and cervical swabs will identify common infections and may be more conveniently undertaken in general practice. This does not preclude referral to the GUM clinic.

Sexually transmitted infections (STIs)

Chlamydia trachomatis

Chlamydia is an extremely common cause of infertility, associated with pelvic inflammatory disease and blocked fallopian tubes (Owen 1993). As the infection is usually asymptomatic it may go undetected for many years. Often the only time the infection, or its antibodies, are detected is when the woman either presents to her GP with pelvic inflammatory disease or because she is unable to conceive.

Chlamydia infection is transferred through vaginal delivery, and can result in conjunctivitis in the neonate, leading to corneal scarring and blindness, and pneumonia caused by inhalation of infected material during delivery (Edwards 1999). Although easily treated with antibiotics, a woman with a positive result should be referred to the GUM clinic for contact tracing of partners, and screening for concurrent infections.

Syphilis and gonorrhoea

The incidence of syphilis rose 37% between 2003 and 2004, while cases of gonorrhoea dropped 11% (Health Protection Agency (HPA) 2005). Once thought easily treated, gonorrhoea is now reported to becoming resistant to antibiotic treatment (HPA 2005). Undetected and untreated infection may result in transplacental infection of the fetus.

Cytomegalovirus (CMV)

CMV affects most people, with 90% of infections being asymptomatic, and 20–30% of cases occurring in the first year of life.

Following a primary infection the virus can become latent and can be reactivated at a later date should the immune system become compromised.

Transmission of this virus can be via droplet, body secretions, sexual transmission, transplacental or via breast milk (NHS Direct 2006). Infection during early pregnancy can lead to miscarriage or the baby being born deaf. CMV is a major cause of fever-induced seizure in babies.

Maternal infection does not always cause congenital infections, although there is a 25–50% transmission rate during a primary maternal infection to the fetus (Fowler et al. 1992). Unlike damage due to rubella infections, there does not appear to be a relationship between gestational age and fetal damage due to CMV.

HIV

In England and Scotland an estimated 0.1% of women had undiagnosed HIV prior to antenatal testing (HPA 2005). One in every 534 women giving birth in 2004 was HIV infected. The greatest prevalence is in women born in sub-Saharan Africa, Central America and the Caribbean. Diagnosis and treatment prior to pregnancy will reduce transmission to an infant.

Women who are positive to, or at risk of contracting, any STI should be made aware of the risks of transmission and given appropriate advice, preferably by staff at a GUM clinic. Women attending specialist clinics can access expert advice, treatment and a confidential contact tracing service.

Group B Streptococcus

Although Group B Streptococcus (GBS) is carried asymptomatically by women and requires no treatment, it causes neonatal infection in one to three of 1000 live births, causing lethal bacterial infection in the infant (Read 2003). GBS in pregnancy is associated with:

- late miscarriage
- stillbirth
- pre-term labour and delivery
- premature delivery
- neonatal infection. (Owen 1993; Read 2003)

Genetic disorders

Genetic disorders may result from single gene disorders, chromosomal abnormalities or congenital malformations such as neural tube defects, although many abnormal babies are born to healthy people with no known risk factors. Approximately 2–3% of women are at high or recurrent risk of their child having an inherited disorder (Office of Population Censuses and Surveys 1994).

The House of Commons Health Committee (1991) acknowledged a need for improved genetic screening. A complete medical family history will help to identify those at risk of an inherited disorder. This includes partners who are first cousins, or those who may carry a dominantly inherited genetic defect.

Haemaglobinopathies will identify single gene disorders such as beta-thalassaemia (Mediterranean origin), sickle cell abnormalities (Afro-Caribbean origin), and Tay Sachs Disease (Ashkenazi Jewish origin). The identification of a disorder, screening for confirmation and referral for appropriate counselling will provide optimum care for both parent and baby.

Maternity units will advise on local referral procedures for genetic counselling.

Women with diabetes mellitus

Poor glycaemic control in early pregnancy in women with pre-existing diabetes mellitus (DM) results in a higher incidence of congenital malformation and spontaneous abortions. About 6–9% of babies born to women with DM have a major congenital malformation, compared with 2–3% of the general population, but fewer than half of women with DM plan their pregnancies (Kendrick 2004). As well as the above pre-conception advice, these women should be referred to the secondary care multidisciplinary team as soon as the pregnancy is confirmed to try to obtain the lowest possible HBAIc without significant episodes of hypoglycaemia.

Practice nurse role in preconception care

A community profile will highlight specific areas of pre-conceptional need. These may include data about teenage conceptions, babies born with neural tube defects, low birth weight babies, drug abusers or the level of sexually transmitted infections in the locality. There are several areas in which the practice nurse has a key role in promoting pre-conceptional health (Box 4.6). This role should complement, rather than compete with, advice given by a midwife or other specialist agencies.

Prevention and management of osteoporosis

Osteoporosis is a silent disease that is often unrecognised until the sufferer experiences pain from a fracture. It is accepted as a female disease occurring post-menopause, but can also affect men and pre-menopausal women, and can be related to many other conditions other than simple oestrogen deficiency at menopause.

The disease process of osteoporosis will be examined in order to enable the reader to identify areas where health promotion may be appropriate in

---

Box 4.6   The practice nurse role in preconception care

- Check rubella status, give MMR if required, advise to avoid pregnancy for 1 month post-vaccine
- Advise folic acid supplements while trying to conceive and for first 12 weeks of pregnancy, with increased dietary folates: reinforce with leaflet
- Advise both prospective parents about the dangers of alcohol, smoking and illicit drugs on both fertility and pregnancy
- Offer screening to exclude chlamydia and Group B Streptococcus
- Refer to genito-urinary clinic if appropriate
- Assess need for genetic counselling or specialist support. Liaise with midwife and refer as necessary
- Advise on all aspects of general healthy lifestyle

---

their working environment. This is essential in order to maximise bone density for vulnerable groups and delay the onset of this condition. Medical management will be mentioned only where appropriate.

Definition

Osteoporosis is a systemic disease characterised by low bone mass, micro-architectural deterioration of bone tissue, and consequent skeletal fragility, with an increase in fracture risk (World Health Organisation 1994, cited in Arthur & Hill 2006, p 67).

Bone formation

Several hormones control the formation, resorption and repair of bone (Figure 4.4). Calcitonin stops osteoclasts dissolving bone when high calcium level in the blood. Vitamin D increases calcium absorption from food in the gut, and plays an important part in bone formation. Parathyroid hormone maintains level of calcium in the blood and also acts on the kidneys, reducing the loss of calcium in the urine and increasing absorption of calcium from food in the gut The sex hormones allow bone cells to respond fully to the other major controlling hormones. The maximum growth spurt for girls is 11–15 years, slightly later for boys, while peak bone mass is usually achieved by the age of 30 (Peel & Eastell 1996).

Human bone is continually being resorbed and reformed, with about 10% of the adult skeleton being remodelled each year (Peel & Eastell 1996); bone loss results from an imbalance between resorption and formation. After skeletal maturity, bone is lost in both sexes at about 1% a year, although women have an accelerated bone loss for 5–10 years post menopause.

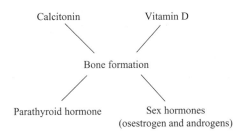

Figure 4.4 Hormone influences in bone formation (Dixon & Woolf 1989).

However, some elderly people show no signs of bone loss (Swedish Council on Technology Assessment in Health Care 1997).

Epidemiology

An estimated 1.2 million women in the United Kingdom have osteoporosis. One in two women and one in five men aged over 50 years will suffer a fracture, with a lifetime risk of fracture in women at age 50 being greater than breast cancer or cardiovascular disease (NOS 2006a). Riggs and Melton (1995) reported 10–20% mortality over the subsequent six months following a hip fracture, 50% of sufferers being unable to walk without help, and 25% requiring long term domiciliary care. The cost of treating all osteoporotic fractures in post-menopausal women has been predicted to increase to more than £2.1 billion by 2010 (National Osteoporosis Society 2006a).

Classification of osteoporosis

Postmenopausal osteoporosis results from accelerated bone loss, probably as a result of oestrogen deficiency. Typically, women in their 60s and 70s present with distal forearm fractures and crushed lumbar or thoracic vertebra. The latter is the most common osteoporotic fracture. Other less common sites are the humerus, ribs and pelvis.

Senile osteoporosis results from the slower age related bone loss that occurs in men and women, typically manifesting at the femoral neck.

Secondary osteoporosis is related to other diseases, particularly those affecting absorption of calcium, immobility and eating disorders (see Box 4.7).

Risk factors

The two main factors that determine whether or not a woman will develop osteoporosis are the peak pre-menopausal adult bone mass and the rate of post-menopausal bone loss. The main risk factors are listed in Table 4.3, and the protective factors are listed in Box 4.8.

Box 4.7   Secondary diseases as causes of osteoporosis

(Cohen, Lancman, Mogul, Marks & Smith 1997; Dennison & Cooper 1996; Peel & Eastell 1996; National Osteoporosis Society 2006a; Rosen 1997)

- Hyperthyroidism*
- Diabetes*
- Malabsorption
- Chronic liver disease
- Ischaemic heart disease
- Systemic lupus erythematosus
- Epilepsy**
- Rheumatoid arthritis
- Myeloma
- Anorexia

*The correction of hypo or hyperfunction of an endocrine gland can increase bone mineral density
**Medication can adversely affect bone metabolism

Endocrine disorders are the most frequent cause of secondary osteoporosis, while the risk to patients on long-term corticosteroids, including those with rheumatoid arthritis, brittle asthma and systemic lupus erythematosus cannot be overstated. Patients prescribed 7.5 mg or more of daily prednisolone have over a 50% increased risk of non-vertebral fractures in the first year of treatment (National Osteoporosis Society 2006b).

Young amenorrhoeic women may lose as much as 2–6% of their bone mass each year. Women who have used long-acting intra-muscular contraception tend to have a lower bone mineral density than women who have not, with the effects on bone being greatest in the first 2–3 years of use (Medicines and Healthcare Products Regulatory Agency 2004). Other hormonal treatments such as for epilepsy exacerbate this risk (Medical and Healthcare Regulatory Agency 2003).

Activity 4.3

Referring to Table 4.3, identify your practice population that is at risk of osteoporosis. Consider local demography, including age and socio-economic distribution, and secondary factors. Raise these figures at a practice team meeting for discussion and possible action plan.

Table 4.3 Risk factors for osteoporosis

Factor	Rationale
Being female	1 in 3 women will suffer an osteoporosis fracture at some time in their lives
Being a smoker	May lead to early menopause and oestrogen deficiency
High alcohol consumption	Suppresses bone formation and may lead to hypogonadism
Prolonged inactivity/immobility	Weight = bearing exercise stengthens bone
Thin frame	May fail to achieve peak bone mass
Genetics	Genetic factors may account for up to 70% of the variability in peak bone mass
Hypogonadism	Androgens necessary for bone formation
Race	Being white or oriental increases risk
Corticosteroids	Those on long-term oral steroids (7.5 mg day), e.g. for brittle asthma
Oestrogen deficiency	Amenorrhoea of more than six months. May be due to natural causes or due to being underweight, anorexia or excessive exercise, or from treatment for endometriosis. Or from injectable contraceptive
Age	An accelerated rate of bone loss occurs following menopause, with 50% of a woman's bone mass being lost by the age of 75 years
Premature menopause	Under 40 years of age or hysterectomy before the menopause

Data from: Dennison & Cooper 1996; Hill 2006; National Osteoporosis Society 2006a; Peel & Eastell 1996; Rosen 1997; Segal & Lane 1997; Stevenson 1995)

Box 4.8   Factors protecting against osteoporosis (Dixon & Woolf 1989)

Early menarche, before the age of 13
Late menopause, after the age of 55
Having had several children
Breastfeeding
Taking the oral contraceptive pill
Non-smoker
Being overweight
Being active from childhood
Being well nourished as a child, with a high calcium intake

Secondary causes

The monitoring and correction of an underlying secondary cause, such as hypo or hyper function of endocrine diseases such as thyroid disorders and diabetes, can increase bone mineral density (Rosen 1997). A simple audit and protocol could redress any deficiencies in current management (see Chapter 2).

Identification of at-risk patients

People at risk of osteoporosis may be identified through a disease register/ computer analysis of diagnosis and/or medication. Routine height checks give only a rough estimate of possible risk, and have limited value in establishing the level of bone density in an individual (Swedish Council on Technology Assessment in Health Care 1997), but may identify people with height loss who should be referred for further assessment. Immobile patients in nursing and residential homes are at increased risk, and should be assessed. It may be useful to devise a protocol for practice use, to ensure all the doctors and nurses use the same criteria. Nurses must also be alert for young women with secondary amenorrhoea, whatever the cause. Women may require advice on alternative methods of contraception (see risk factors above).

Prevention of osteoporosis through health promotion

Although the terms health promotion and health education are often used interchangeably, McKnight and Edwards (1998) make the point that health promotion can appear coercive and aggressive, instead of merely educative. You may wish to bear this in mind when planning any health promotion activities.

Most of the data on osteoporosis involves post-menopausal women, as they are the largest at-risk group for this disease. It has been noted above, however, that there are a range of at-risk groups for which health education and health promotion is essential.

The National Dairy Council (NDC) highlighted calcium intake to be inversely related to social class, with lone mothers having significantly lower dietary calcium (NDC 1996). Slimmers also have a tendency to reduce their dairy, and therefore their calcium, intake which compromises their skeletal health. This suggests that health promotion must not focus on middle-aged and elderly women (recognised women at risk), but on the whole female population.

The author assumes that the reader already undertakes health promotion using poster displays, leaflets, one-to-one counselling and groupwork. Other methods, such as community initiatives are more difficult to organise, and require the commitment of several health disciplines, or associated agencies. However, these initiatives are challenging, target a wider audience and can be worth the effort.

The different models of health promotion are not discussed, but their theories are implicitly incorporated into general healthcare, which will relate to primary, secondary and tertiary prevention (Naidoo & Wills 2000).

Primary health prevention (A): aims to prevent the onset of osteoporosis, and may relate to all age groups.

Secondary prevention (B): involves alleviating pain and reducing further fractures once osteoporosis is established.

Tertiary prevention (C): refers to assisting people with chronic or irreversible ill health cope with their condition and maximise their health potential. Multiple osteoporotic vertebral crush fractures lead to severe kyphosis, which is irreversible.

Health promotion for each of the three stages of health prevention overlap – these stages are referred to as A, B or C in the following text for convenience.

Children and young women

The National Dairy Council (2006) discusses the need to prevent osteoporosis by promoting a calcium-rich diet and healthy lifestyle from childhood. Smoking, excess alcohol consumption and excess salt intake (from salty snacks and processed foods) are detrimental to the skeleton, but are commonly a daily part of the teenage lifestyles.

One health promotion strategy to maximise peak bone mass in girls involved a multi-disciplinary approach (Figure 4.5) (Edwards 1997). Although the girls did not appear to increase their dietary calcium intake, the campaign reached other vulnerable groups and raised general awareness of diet and physical activity related to bone health. Simple areas to address include walking to school when possible and substituting milk for sugary drinks.

Teenagers are often unreceptive to health promotion, so health promotion (A) must target children and their parents to achieve maximum peak bone mass to promote strong bones that will last a lifetime. Soft drinks and convenience foods should be avoided as they often contain large amounts of phosphorus that leads to loss of calcium from bone (Osteoporosis Treatment 2006). The School Food Trust (2006) has advised the government that schools should stop selling confectionary, crisps and fizzy drinks to improve

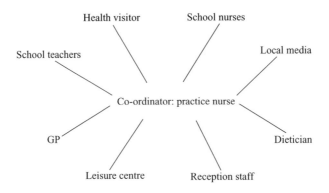

Figure 4.5 Multi-disciplinary approach to health promotion. This approach utilises the expertise and knowledge of each discipline and improves overall awareness within the community.

children's health. This may be a step in increasing bone mineral density in young people.

Vegans

Vegan diets are often high in roughage, which may hinder calcium absorption from other foods. This is also relevant when people are encouraged to eat a low fat, high fibre diet. It is essential to assess any diet for adequate calcium intake as calcium supplements may sometimes be necessary (A, B, C). A dietician will usually be willing to offer advice.

Exercise

Physical activity can delay the progression of osteoporosis by slowing the reduction of bone mineral density from the late 20s upwards (National Osteoporosis Society 2006a). It has been suggested that incidence of osteoporosis is increasing due to decreased physical activity, as well as increasing longevity (Arthur & Hill 2006).

Regular physical activity has a beneficial effect on the skeleton, and should be encouraged from an early age (A). Bone is strengthened through weight bearing exercises such as walking, dancing and aerobics, although excessive exercise can have an adverse effect on bone growth. Other benefits of exercise include improved balance, which reduces accidents and falls (B, C), and improved general well-being.

Health promotion must be targeted to need. In areas with low car ownership, children may well take plenty of exercise so emphasis will lie on other areas of health. The 'school run' has resulted in fewer children walking to school, as parents fear for their child's safety. Some schools have implemented a 'walking bus' where children walk from a car park or their homes to school under supervision. This is a good example of a community health initiative. For optimal protection, weight-bearing exercise should be maintained throughout life, for men and women (National Osteoporosis Society 2006a; Prodigy 2006b).

Alcohol

Alcohol damages bone cells and reduces calcium absorption. An alcohol intake of more than two units per day increases the risk of an osteoporotic fracture (National Osteoporosis Society 2006a). Health promotion should include advice on alcohol consumption, and support, for women of all ages (A, B, C).

Smoking

Smokers have a significantly increased risk of having a fracture (National Osteoporosis Society 2006a).

Maintaining bone strength

It is essential to maintain any remaining bone through dietary calcium and vitamin D synthesis (B, C). Advice on eating small meals often will reduce discomfort from the abdominal distension that often accompanies kyphosis.

A balanced diet provides all the vitamins and minerals required to develop and maintain strong bones. The recommended daily intake (RDI) for calcium in adults is 700 mg (National Osteoporosis Society 2006a), with 1500 mg a day for postmenopausal women and elderly people (Department of Health 2003). Vitamin D is necessary for calcium absorption for bone formation, which may be obtained from sunlight on the skin. However above the age of 65 there is a four-fold decrease in the capacity of the skin to produce Vitamin D. The RDI of Vitamin D for this group is 400 IU (Prodigy 2006b), although a level of 400–800 IU has been quoted (Stott 2006). This information can be promoted through simple dietary advice during any consultation, supported by literature if appropriate.

Weight bearing exercise should also be encouraged. People with spinal osteoporosis (B, C) are encouraged to exercise to improve posture, balance and breathing (Dixon & Woolf 1989). A physiotherapist may be willing to offer advice for a specific client.

Accident prevention

The risk of falls increases with alcohol consumption, while an increased risk of falls in epileptic patients can be related to drug toxicity (Cohen et al. 1997). Drug regimes in these patients, and for those where multiple drugs are prescribed, may need reviewing by the doctor. Patients who are prescribed hypnotics, sedatives and hypertensive treatments are at an increased risk of falling. Advice on falls prevention should be considered when reviewing their medication. Some localities have exercise on referral schemes where people can have an individually tailored exercise programme; this may improve balance and reduce falls for some patients.

Osteoporosis in men

Osteoporotic fractures in men occur most commonly at the hip, usually the result of some other condition or treatment such as immobility or corticosteroid therapy, although hypogonadism is reported to be a major risk factor for osteoporosis in men (National Osteoporosis Society 2005). An increase in bone formation and decrease in resorption can be achieved with testosterone treatment in men with hypogonadism. Nurses may be involved in treatment compliance and offering support for these men.

Management of established osteoporosis

The goals of treatment for patients with established osteoporosis are to:

- maintain normal bone
- to prevent the deterioration of normal bone to osteoporotic bone.

Medication

The aim of drug treatment is to prevent a first osteoporotic fracture in those with osteoporosis, and to reduce further fractures in those who have already suffered one. Drugs used to treat established osteoporosis prevent further bone loss and can reduce the risk of further fractures by up to 50% (see Box 4.9).

HRT is no longer considered the first line of treatment for osteoporosis in women over 50 years because of increased risks of breast cancer and the potential risks of cardiovascular disease (MHRA 2003). HRT is classed as a second-line treatment for osteoporosis, but is still prescribed for women who

> **Box 4.9 Medication to treat established osteoporosis (National Institute for Clinical Excellence 2005b; National Osteoporosis Society 2006b; Peel & Eastell 1996)**
>
> These include:
>
> 1. Calcium and Vitamin D supplements are reported to be useful in elderly patients, but are probably inefffective in perimenopausal women.
> 2. Calcitonin is an antiresorptive hormone, usually given with calcium and vitamin D, to prevent bone loss and may lead to an increase in bone density. This is useful as a short-term treatment after spinal fracture.
> 3. Biphosphonates reduce osteoclast activity (breakdown of bone), and increase vertebral bone mineral density. This then lowers the risk of vertebral crush fractures.
> 4. Raloxifene – may be used when biphosphates are unsuitable for any reason.
> 5. Teriparatide – used for women aged over 65 years for whom biphosphanates are unsuitable or have not worked.
> 6. Hormone replacement therapy is not a first line treatment, but may be useful for menopausal symptoms with bone protection back up.
>
> The reader is referred to the British National Formulary for details of the above drugs.

have had a early menopause (before aged 45) until they reach the average age of menopause (National Osteoporosis Society 2006b).

Calcium and Vitamin D is commonly used to prevent osteoporosis, while NICE guidance recommends biphosphonates as first-line therapy for most patients with established osteoporosis (National Institute for Clinical Excellence 2005a).

Analgesia

Long-term analgesia may be required to control the pain in established osteoporosis (B, C). Exercises to improve posture may alleviate some pain, while referral to a physiotherapist for alternative methods of pain relief, such as electrical stimulation (TENS) may be helpful. If a patient has uncontrolled pain, the nurse may need to act as the patient's advocate and refer back to doctor for review of pain control (see Chapter 1).

Box 4.10   How to encourage concordance with treatments

- Assess concordance during consultations – may attend for another reasons.
- Does she understand why she is taking the treatment?
- How often she should take it?
- Ask about side effects.
- Support information with literature from the National Osteoporosis Society, or refer to website.
- May prefer an alternative method - refer to GP.

Concordance with treatment (A, B, C)

It is essential that patients be empowered to be concordant with their treatment (Box 4.10). Nurses have a key role in encouraging concordance, or suggesting an alternative method of delivery. Regular follow-ups with the nurse allows the patient to discuss any concerns, may lead to improved levels of concordance, and offers opportunities to discuss any other related health issues such as diet, smoking cessation and exercise. Cooper (2006) reported that the reasons why women stop treatment are usually related to side effects or because they are asymptomatic. Nurse-led patient support improves persistence.

Activity 4.4

Devise a health promotion strategy to maintain bone strength for men and women with established osteoporosis.

Summary

Epidemiological studies are the key to assessing health needs. They can be used to examine local, national and international problems; show changing health trends and disease patterns; and identify groups of people within a community who may be at risk from conditions likely to affect their health and well-being. Practice nurses are important members of the primary healthcare team that can assess and prioritise healthcare needs in the community. The key issue is that when you have identified a need, are there resources to deal with it?

Pre-conception is the ideal opportunity for a risk assessment of couples planning a pregnancy. Pre-conceptual counselling enables women and men to prepare for pregnancy and make informed choices surrounding conception and pregnancy (Prodigy 2006a). The practice nurse, in planned and opportunistic consultations, can carry out efficient, effective and appropriate health education.

As demography changes with increased longevity, the morbidity and mortality of osteoporosis is also set to increase. Nurses must use their excellent communication skills to identify people at risk of osteoporosis and promote the benefits of a healthy lifestyle to reduce premature bone loss.

It is important to determine the level of service the practice wishes to offer. Is this a proactive approach to prevent disease, or a reactive approach to treat a condition? The latter offers easily accessible quantifiable data, whereas the results of the former will not be apparent for many years.

Although the cost effectiveness of primary health prevention cannot be measured for many years, nurses have the resources (themselves) to promote health from the pre-conception to the grave.

Key points

- Need can be normative, felt, expressed or comparative.
- Needs assessments assures appropriate allocation of resources.
- Community profiles are a means to assess local healthcare needs.
- The health of both prospective parents is important for a healthy baby.
- Effective health promotion can delay the onset of osteoporosis in both men and women.
- Health promotion can improve compliance with management of established disease.

Recommended reading

Buttriss J, Wynne A & Stanner S (2001) *Nutrition. A Handbook for Community Nurses.* London: Whurr.
Includes recommendations for nutrition throughout life.
Hill J (2006) *Rheumatology Nursing. A Creative Approach, 2nd edn.* Chichester: Wiley.
For detailed information on osteoporosis.
Naidoo J & Wills J (2000) *Health Promotion. Foundations for Practice 2nd edn.* London: Bailliere Tindall.
An excellent health promotion text.

References

Arthur V & Hill J (2006) The musculoskeletal system and the rheumatic diseases. In J Hill J (Ed.) *Rheumatology Nursing. A Creative Approach, 2nd edn.* Chichester: Wiley.

Bernard M and Meade K (1993) *Women Come of Age.* London: Edward Arnold.

Billingham K (1994) Beyond the individual. *Health Visitor* 67(9), 295.

Billings JR & Cowley S (1995) Approaches to community needs assessment: a literature review. *Journal of Advanced Nursing* 22, 721–730.

Blaxter M (1990) *Health and Lifestyles.* London: Tavistock/Routledge.

Bradshaw JS (1972) A taxonomy of social need. In G McLachlan (Ed.) *Problems and Progress in Medical Care: Essays on Current Research, 7th series.* London: Oxford University Press.

British Nutrition Foundation (2002) *Folate for the Family.* (CG 41). www.nutrition.org.uk/home (accessed 18 August 2006).

British Nutrition Foundation (2006) *Folate and Health.* www.nutrition.org.uk/home (accessed 12 September 2007).

Buttriss J, Wynne A & Stanner S (2001) *Nutrition. A Handbook for Community Nurses.* London: Whurr.

Centers for Disease Control and Prevention (2006) *Toxoplasmosis: An Important Message for Women.* www.cdc.gov/ncidod/dpd/parasites/toxoplasmosis/Toxowomen (accessed 18 August 2006).

Cohen A, Lancman M, Mogul H, Marks S & Smith K (1997) Strategies to protect bone mass in the older patient with epilepsy. *Geriatrics* 52(8), 70,75–78,81.

Cooper A (2006) Tackling compliance issues in osteoporosis treatment. *Independent Nurse* 6–19 November, 26

Crawley H (1993) Plan before conception for a healthy pregnancy. *Mimms Magazine Weekly* 19 January, 24–29.

Day NL, Jasperse D & Richardson G (1989) Prenatal exposure to alcohol: effect on infant growth and morphological characteristics. *Paediatrics* 84, 536–541.

Dennison E & Cooper C (1996) The epidemiology of osteoporosis. *British Journal of Clinical Practice* 50(1), 33–36.

Department of Health (1990) *NHS and Community Care Act.* London: HMSO.

Department of Health (1992) *The Health of the Nation: a Strategy for Health in England.* Cm 1986 London: HMSO.

Department of Health (1995) *Variations in Health.* London: HMSO.

Department of Health (2000) *Report on Folic acid and its role in the reduction of Neural tube defects published by Coma.* London: COMA

Department of Health (2003) *Further advice on safety of HRT.* www.dh.gov.uk

Department of Health (2006a) *PCT and SHA roles and functions.* www.dh.gov.uk/PublicationsAndStatistics (accessed 26 August 2006).

Department of Health (2006b) *General Question and Answer on Practice Based Commissioning.* www.dh.gov.uk/PolicyAndGuidance/OrganisationalPolicy (accessed 26 August 2006).

Department of Health (2006c) *National Service Frameworks (NSF's).* www.dh.gov.uk/PolicyAndGuidance/HealthAndSocialCareTopics (accessed 26 August 2006).

Department of Health (2006d) *Priorities and Planning Framework for 2003–2006*. www. Department of Health.gov.uk/PolicyAndGuidance/HealthAndSocialCareTopics (accessed 26 August 2006).

Department of Health (2006e) *Folic Acid – What all Women Should Know*. London: HMSO.

Department of Health (2006f) *Immunisation Against Infectious Disease, 3rd edn*. London: The Stationary Office.

Department of Health (2007) *Alcohol and Pregnancy*. www.dh.gov.uk (accessed 12 September 2007).

Department of Health and Social Security (1990) *Vitamin A and Pregnancy. Letter from the Chief Medical and Nursing Officers* DL/CMO(90)11, PL/CNO(90)10. London: DOH.

Diabetes UK (2006) *Pregnancy and Diabetes*. www.diabetesuk.org.uk/pregnancy (accessed 27 August 2006).

Dixon A & Woolf A (1989) *Avoiding Osteoporosis*. London: Macdonald and Co.

Economides D & Braithwaite J (1994) Smoking, pregnancy and the fetus. *Journal Royal Society Health* 114, 198–201.

Edwards M (1997) A strategy to maximise peak bone mass. *1996 NDC/RCGP Practice Team Nutrition Award*. Unpublished.

Edwards M (1999) Your role in the management of chlamydia. *Practice Nurse* 18(5), 293–294, 297.

Edwards M (2006) Preconception care. *Practice Nurse* 32(2), 43, 45–46.

Ernhart CB, Sokol RJ, Martier S, Moran E, Nadler D, Ager JW & Wolf A (1987) Alcohol teratogenicity in the human: a detailed assessment of specificity, critical period, and threshold *American Journal of Obstetrics and Gynecology* 156, 33–39.

Farmer R, Miller D & Lawrenson R (1996) *Lecture Notes on Epidemiology and Public Health Medicine 4th edn*. Oxford: Blackwell Science.

Fowler KB, Stagno PHS, Pass RF, Britt WJ, Boll TJ & Alford CA (1992) The outcome of congenital cytomegalovirus infection in relation to maternal antibody status. *New England Journal of Medicine* 325, 663–667.

Griffiths-Jones A (1997) Tuberculosis in homeless people. *Nursing Times* 93(9), 60–61.

Harris A (1996) What is a primary care-led policy? In P Littlejohns & C Victor (Eds) *Making Sense of a Primary Care-led Health Service*. Oxford: Radcliffe Medical Press.

Health Protection Agency (2005) *Mapping the Issues. HIV and Other Sexually Transmitted Infections in the UK: 2005*. www.hpa.org.uk (accessed 18August 2006).

Henderson S (1995) *Drug Information for Women: Drugs and Your Health*. London: ISSD.

Hill J (2006) *Rheumatology Nursing. A Creative Approach, 2nd edn*. Chichester: Wiley.

House of Commons Health Committee (1991) *Maternity Services: Preconception. The Fourth Report*. London: HMSO.

Keen J & Alison LH (2001) Drug misusing parents: key points for health professionals. *Archives Disease in Childhood* 85, 296–299.

Kendrick J (2004) Preconception care of women with diabetes. *The Journal of Perinatal and Neonatal Nursing* (18)1, 14–27.

Leuzzi RA & Scoles KS (1996) Preconception counselling for the primary care physician. *Medical Clinics of North America* 80(2), 337–374.

McKnight S & Edwards M (1998) Health promotion In C Blackie (Ed.) *Community Health Care Nursing*. Edinburgh: Churchill Livingstone.

Medicine and Healthcare Regulatory Agency and the Committee on Safety of Medicines (2003) *Hormone Replacement Therapy: Latest Safety Update*. December. www.mhra.gov.uk (accessed 12 September 2007).

Medicines and Healthcare Products Regulatory Agency (2004) *Questions and Answers Related to the Effect of Depo-Provera on Bones*. www.mhra.gov.uk (accessed 18 August 2006).

Medical Research Council Vitamin Study Group (1991) Prevention of neural tube defects: Results of the Medical Research Council Vitamin Study. *Lancet* 238, 131–137.

Moos MK (2004) Preconceptional health promotion: progress in changing a prevention paradigm. *The Journal of Perinatal and Neonatal Nursing* 18(1), 2–13.

Naidoo J & Wills J (2000) *Health Promotion. Foundations for Practice 2nd edn*. London: Bailliere Tindall.

National Dairy Council (1996) *Calcium and Bone Health Topical Update 7* London: National Dairy Council.

National Dairy Council (2006) *Bone Health and Osteoporosis*. www.nationaldairycouncil. org.uk (accessed 18 August 2006).

NHS Direct (2006) *Cytomegalovirus*. www.nhsdirect.nhs.uk (accessed 26 August 2006).

National Institute for Clinical Excellence (2005a) *NICE Technology Appraisal: Strontium Review*. www.nice.org.uk (accessed 27 August 2006).

National Institute for Clinical Excellence (2005b) *Osteoporosis – Secondary Prevention*. TA087. London: NICE.

National Osteoporosis Society (2005) *Information sheet on Testosterone and Osteoporosis*. www.nos.org.uk (accessed 27 August 2006).

National Osteoporosis Society (2006a) *Osteoporosis Facts and Figures* V1.1. www.nos. org.uk (accessed 28 August 2006).

National Osteoporosis Society (2006b) FAQs about bone health. *Practice Nurse* 31(4), 55–56.

Office for National Statistics (1997) *Social Trends 27*. London: The Stationery Office.

Office of Population Censuses and Surveys (1994) *Congenital Malformations Statistics: Notifications 1992 Series MB3(8)*. London: HMSO.

Osteoporosis Treatment (2006) *Calcium and Osteoporosis*. www.osteoporosistreatment. co.uk (accessed 28 August 2006).

Owen P (1993) Vaginal Discharge. In A McPherson (Ed.) *Women's Problems in General Practice*. Oxford: Oxford University Press.

Peel N & Eastell R (1996) Osteoporosis. In M Snaith (Ed.) *ABC of Rheumatology* London: BMJ Publishing Group.

Prodigy (2006a) *Preconceptual Counselling. Patient Information Sheet*. www.prodigy.nhs. uk (accessed 31 August 2006).

Prodigy (2006b) *Osteoporosis. Patient information sheet*. www.prodigy.nhs.uk (accessed 31 August 2006).

Read S (2003) Group B Streptococcus: testing and treatment. *British Journal of Midwifery* 11(3), 160–163.

Riggs BL & Melton LJ (1995) The worldwide problem of osteoporosis: insights afforded by epidemiology. *Bone* 17(5 Suppl), 505S–511S.

Rolater S, Winslow E & Jaconson AF (2000) One drink too many. *American Journal of Nursing* 100(5), 64–66.

Rosen CJ (1997) Endocrine disorders and osteoporosis. *Current Opinion in Rheumatology* 9(4), 355–361.

Schoendorf KC & Kiely JL (1992) Relationship of sudden infant death syndrome to maternal smoking during and after pregnancy. *Paediatrics* 90, 905–908.

School Food Trust (2006) *Transforming School Food*. www.schoolfoodtrust.org.uk (accessed 12 September 2007).

Segal LG & Lane NE (1997) Osteoporosis and systemic lupus erythematosus: etiology and treatment strategies. *Annales de Medecine Interne* 147(4), 281–289.

Stevenson JC (1995) The impact of bone loss in women with endometriosis. *International Journal of Gynaecology and Obstetrics* 50(Suppl 1), S11–15.

Stott P (2006) Managing postmenopausal osteoporosis in general practice (interactive case history). *BMJ Learning* www.bmjlearning.com (accessed 13 September 2006).

Swedish Council on Technology Assessment in Healthcare (1997) Bone density measurement – a systematic review. A review from SBU, the Swedish Council on Technology Assessment in Health Care. *Journal of Internal Medicine* 739(Suppl), 1–60.

Tudor Hart J (1971) The inverse care law. *Lancet* 1, 405–412.

Vallance P (1996) Drugs and the fetus. *British Medical Journal* 312, 1053–1054.

Verbiest S (2005) Folic acid fortification. Should oral contraceptives be next?: PRO. *The American Journal of Maternal/Child Nursing* 30(4), 228.

World Health Organisation (1978) *Primary Health Care: Report of the International Conference on Primary Health Care, Alma-Ata, USSR, 6–12 September 1978*. Geneva: World Health Organisation.

Wynn M & Wynn A (1991) *The Case for Preconception Care of Men and Women*. Oxford: AB Academic Publishers.

Useful addresses

British Nutrition Foundation
High Holborn House
52-54 High Holborn
London WC1 V 6RQ
Tel: 020 7404 6504
Email: postbox@nutrition.org.uk
www.nutrition.org.uk

Department of Health
Some documents can be downloaded. Most can be ordered as hard copies.
www.dh.gov.uk

Diabetes UK
For information on diabetes and pregnancy.
www.diabetes.org.uk

The Amarant Trust
Helpline staffed by nurses. Information about problems suffered before,
during and after the menopause. Monday-Friday 11.00-18.00
Tel: 01293 413000
www.amarantmenopause.trust.org.uk

The National Osteoporosis Society
For information on all aspects of osteoporosis in men and women.
Camerton
Bath BA2 0PJ
NOS Helpline Tel: 0845 450 0230
NOS osteoporosis nurses: email: nurses@nos.org.uk
www.nos.org.uk

Centers for Disease Control and Prevention.
Has useful information on toxoplasmosis.
www.cdc.gov/ncidod/dpd/parasites/toxoplasmosis/Toxowomen.

The Toxoplasmosis Trust
The Toxoplasmosis Trust is run by Tommy's the baby charity.
email: mailbox@tommys.org

Chapter 5

Men's Health

Marilyn Edwards and Glenn Turp

Any audit of general practice consultations would confirm that men attend less frequently than women. Mortality figures show that although both genders are living longer, the average men's life expectancy is five years less than women (National Statistics 2006). This chapter examines the social issues surrounding men's health, and tries to identify why men are often reluctant to seek medical advice or accept health education. This is pertinent when planning services and promoting health (see Chapter 4).

There is an assumption that all men are heterosexual unless they state otherwise. The key issues relating to the health of men who have sex with men (MSM) are explored through the male author's experience of working with men and through his own experience; some of this is narrative text. The underlying problems may challenge the reader's current thinking about this topic, and make their service inclusive to MSM. Testicular and prostate cancer have been included in this chapter to highlight the nurse's role in promoting health and encouraging men to seek medical advice at an early stage of a disease process. Although early detection and treatment of malignancy reduces mortality from testicular cancer, the benefits of prostate screening are controversial. The reader will, however, have the facts to share with men who want information and support about these diseases.

Social issues surrounding men's health

Men are physically more vulnerable than women from the moment they are conceived until they die (Nicholson 1993). Although their health needs are apparently greater than those of women, these appear to be inadequately addressed.

Lloyd (2001) offers three definitions for men's health:

1. men's health is biological, e.g. prostate and testicular cancers, sexually transmitted infections and other sexual health matters

The Informed Practice Nurse, Edwards, M. (2008), Chichester: Wiley.

2. men's health is about risk and risk taking
3. men's health is primarily about masculinity and the impact this process has on the way men perceive their health.

Health is influenced by a combination of biology, personal choice and social factors. Issues relating to inequalities of health are paramount to men's health; those specific to men who have sex with men are covered in the following section of this chapter.

Gender

The higher male mortality may be attributed to physiological sex differences, including a slightly higher risk of birth injury and asphyxia resulting from male babies being on average slightly larger than females, and a higher rate of genetically transmitted disorders (Morgan, Calnan & Manning 1985). Mortality rates for men have remained markedly higher than for females. Life expectancy at birth has increased between 1985 and 2001; for females from 78 to 80.4 years, compared with 72 to 75.7 years for males (Bone, Bebbington, Jagger, Morgan & Nicholaas 1995; National Statistics 2006). Gender is an important determinant of health status and efforts to reduce the inequalities between sexes aims to improve health provision for men (Department of Health 2007).

Health and masculinity

The foundations of masculinity are laid down in boyhood, when boys are socialised into acceptable masculine behaviour. Socialisation is continued through the media, where men are portrayed as heroes and workers, able to cope with everyday stress and to solve their own problems. The male gender role stereotype demands real men to be healthy, strong and self-sufficient; seeking help is a sign of weakness.

Masculine competitive and aggressive characteristics may also predispose men to certain stress-related health problems. A competitive striving personality trait (Type A) is associated with an increased risk of coronary heart disease (Nicholson 1993).

The monotony of work and fear of unemployment, housing problems, poverty and family crises were identified as stressors 20 years ago (Morgan et al. 1985); there is no reason to believe that these stressors are any less significant in 2008.

Married men tend to be healthier and have better jobs than do single men of all ages (Nicholson 1993). Although there appears to be no data on this issue, men co-habiting with a partner of either sex may be included in this category. Risks of premature death from all causes are closely related to marital status, and the loss of a partner through death, separation or divorce, poses important threats to health.

Men in Western societies are brought up to value work as an end to itself and fix their identities around particular occupations, where friendship and financial reward may compensate for the threat of redundancy.

Men's health, social class and culture

Much of the documentation on gender and health relates to the inequalities of health due to social class. Health also affects social mobility, as ill health can result in a drop in social class when job prospects suffer, or the person is unable to work.

The most important factor that determines the way a person deals with a symptom appears to be their internal belief structure about the meaning of symptoms and illness. Health is considered a good quality, and few respondents of one study wanted to say they were anything but healthy (Morgan et al. 1985). Illness is perceived as a state of spiritual or moral malaise. Lower social groups consider only serious conditions as illness. It has been argued that the diseases that cause premature death, in particular heart disease and cancer, are closely linked with male lifestyle in our society (Armstrong 1994).

Cardiovascular disease

Cardiovascular disease is one of the main causes of premature death in the UK (death before the age of 75 years), accounting for 32% of premature deaths in men. Approximately one in five men die from coronary heart disease (CHD); 21% of which suffer premature death. Encouragingly, death rates for people under 65 years have fallen by 44% since 1996, mostly attributed to reductions in smoking. During the 1980s the premature death rate fell across all social groups, but fell faster for nonmanual workers than manual workers and the difference in death rates increased.

Ethnic differences in mortality are reported by the British Heart Foundation (2006). Data from the 1990s show the premature death rate from CHD for South Asian men was 46% higher than average, although the rate for men from the Caribbean and West Africa was about half the average rate. The premature death rate from strokes is more alarming. The rate for West Africans was nearly three times higher, and for Caribbeans it was 68% higher than average.

Lifestyle

Alcohol consumption and cigarette smoking were reported to increase with declining class, especially among men (Townsend, Davidson & Whitehead

1992). This was not supported by an epidemiological study by the Department of Health (1996), which concluded that there was little difference between the proportions of employed and unemployed men who drink over the recommended level of 21 units a week. Alcohol may be a support for men who are reluctant to express their emotional and personal needs or to seek support from each other (Nicholson 1993).

Health and employment

Men are stereotyped into employment categories. Working-class men are employed in heavy, risky jobs, while middle-class men are employed in office, or mental work (Cornwall & Lindisfarne 1994). The hazards of manual work reflected in accidents at work, and work related diseases are well known (Hart 1985; Morgan et al. 1985). These hazards are reflected in the increased morbidity and mortality figures of men, and may contribute to women's increased life expectancy over men.

Men may seek danger money associated with hazardous jobs, work overtime, take a second part-time job, or work in the informal economy where there may be poor health and safety conditions.

Hart (1985) suggests that a stressor such as redundancy reduces the immune system, making the patient more susceptible to illness. The difference in men's ability to cope with stress may be due to lack of material resources and the psychological support that assist coping behaviour.

Unemployment may affect men in one of two ways. For some men, it can result in a feeling of worthlessness and a sense of failure, increasing stress and poverty. For others it may result in a reduction of stress caused by poor working conditions, offer financial gain through redundancy payments and allow more time for leisure activities.

Low income and low self-esteem resulting from unemployment may produce high morbidity and mortality due to mental or physical illness, shortened life and high rates of accidents (Fareed 1994).

Tolson (1987) noted the negative effect of a prolonged period of unemployment on man's self-image, impulsive behaviour and sexual relationship with his wife. Long-term unemployment is a health hazard that must be recognised, with mental health service input offered where appropriate.

Low income, whether from unemployment or low-paid employment, also has an indirect effect on health and diet. The high sugar and low fibre content of diets of social groups IV and V compared with groups I and II were identified as contributing to the higher rates of coronary heart disease among the manual classes (Townsend et al. 1992). Some of the variations may, however, be cultural and not merely due to income.

Healthcare services

The male sex role stereotype to be healthy, strong and self-sufficient results in many men delaying seeking medical aid until they are acutely ill. Men appear to leave health matters unattended for longer than women (Lloyd 2001).

Matz (1993) concluded that to meet the needs of men, an environment must be provided in which men feel safe enough to share their needs and feelings and challenge oppressive aspects of sexism and homophobia. In an ideal world, health promotion, education and support would be taken to the populace, rather than waiting for them to come to us. Walk-in centres may meet the health needs of some men better than their general practice, in terms of flexibility and access.

Access to healthcare and health improvement are included in *Quality and Performance in the NHS* (Department of Health 1999). This should be considered realistically for primary healthcare service provision.

The lower uptake of preventative health services among the manual classes has been explained in terms of their general orientation to the present and unwillingness to consider long-term benefits (Morgan et al. 1985), and is due more to cultural norms and voluntary behaviour choices than to material barriers such as limited access (Fareed 1994; Townsend et al. 1992).

Health checks attract the worried well and comfort the middle classes who can afford to follow a reasonably healthy lifestyle. The inverse care law was discussed in Chapter 4. However, a health project in Glasgow has proved that working-class men can, and do, benefit from healthcare input once they overcome the traditional hard man stereotype (McMillan 1995).

Factors affecting men's decisions not to seek healthcare include the inconvenience of taking time off work for appointments and the potential loss of income from absenteeism, although work related stress and competition to achieve career advancement might place men at particular risk of illness.

The quality of healthcare provision varies between social classes. Whereas middle-class patients usually have high expectations of health outcome and are able to articulate their concerns, members of the lower social groups have shorter consultations and receive less information about their condition, with referrals to specialist care highest among patients in social class I and lowest in social class V (Morgan et al. 1985).

Health promotion is received more readily by the middle classes than manual workers, although the latter are said to be in greater need of lifestyle changes. Hart (1985) attributes this to middle-class socialisation that enables this group to adapt to changes in modern culture. Individuals from lower social classes find it more difficult to modify advice to fit their own perceived needs, since most advice is generally based on the values and beliefs of the middle and upper classes (Tettersell and Luft 1994).

Activity 5.1

Undertake, or refer to, a community/practice profile to identify priority issues for healthcare of men in your practice. Is there a high incidence of premature mortality or morbidity from preventable diseases?

Well men

Wellness is peculiar to the individual and is difficult to define. One person may be in permanent pain, but feel well because he can walk to the shops, while another feels ill because of a headache. As noted in Chapter 4, health prevention may be primary, secondary or tertiary. Primary prevention seeks to prevent the onset of disease through risk reduction, for example preventing hypertension by reducing alcohol consumption. Secondary prevention relates to prevention of progression of a disease process, such as the prescribing of aspirin therapy following a heart attack or stroke. Tertiary health prevention involves measures to maximise health and minimise disability from a disease that cannot be cured. This may include lifestyle advice to stabilise blood sugar levels in diabetic patients.

National Service Frameworks (NSF) include preventative measures in their standards, which if followed are designed to reduce morbidity. For example, Standard One of the NSF for Diabetes (Department of Health 2001) includes developing strategies to reduce the risk of people developing Type 2 diabetes. Reducing obesity, encouraging exercise and following a healthy eating regime are all measures to reduce risks of diabetes. Screening well men with a body mass index over 30 may identify asymptomatic diabetes. If identified at an early stage, complications of the disease may be reduced. As black and minority ethnic groups have a higher incidence of diabetes than the white population (Department of Health 2001), practices with a high ethnic population have a challenge to reduce morbidity and mortality in this group.

Primary healthcare nurses are in an ideal position to offer a holistic approach to health. A well-man health check is an opportunity to offer structured health advice and can be incorporated into almost any consultation.

The benefits of cardiovascular screening and subsequent interventions have been controversial and often negative (Family Heart Study Group 1994; Lindholm et al. 1995; Waller et al. 1990). However, structured health counselling has been shown to be a positive move towards adoption of healthy lifestyle changes by men (Edgar 1992).

The term used to describe a well-man check is irrelevant, but the rationale behind each question or activity must be understood by the nurse and the patient for the intervention to be effective, informed and not merely a data collection activity.

General health checks

A health check allows men the opportunity to discuss any health concern, however apparently insignificant, and is an ideal opportunity to review any chronic disease, such as asthma or diabetes that may save a future appointment. General health issues may include bladder and bowel changes or skin conditions.

Family history is nonmodifiable, but many disease risk factors are modifiable. A healthy lifestyle usually includes nonsmoking, moderate drinking, regular exercise and a healthy balanced diet that maintains a BMI of 20–25. As the high incidence of male obesity has been recognised, with two-thirds of English men having a BMI of more than 25 (World Cancer Research Fund 2005), tailored interventions to motivate men to a healthy lifestyle are essential.

The World Cancer Research Fund (2005) advocate moderate activity for at least an hour a day, with vigorous activity for a further hour a week. Men in sedentary occupations can be encouraged to go for a walk at lunchtimes, walk to the paper shop or take a brisk walk after tea. Manual workers often take sufficient unstructured exercise within their work to meet the recommendations. Exercise on referral may be an option for those who would benefit from a structured exercise regime although this may not be available in all localities.

Smoking cessation is integral to the CHD NSF (Department of Health 2000a). This is an area where all health professionals can continue to offer advice and support, referring to a specialist smoking cessation advisor where appropriate (Department of Health 2003).

The Office for National Statistics (1995) reported that the majority of men find health professional advice about alcohol intake helpful but that few men are offered advice. The fear of losing a driving licence and/or employment following a drink-driving incident can be a major incentive to modify alcohol intake. Men with an acknowledged drink problem may wish to be referred

---

Box 5.1   Factors to consider when assessing health

Factor	Risk
Family history	CHD, diabetes, familial hyperlipidaemia
Occupation	unemployed
	stressed – fear of redundancy or high powered job
	skin cancer from working outdoors; travel health, including sexual health (see below)
	chemicals
	hepatitis A or B
	other risks included triggers for asthma, latex allergy, dermatitis;
	hearing loss
Use of recreational drugs	addiction , mental health
Hypertension	CHD, stroke
Diet	affects all aspects of health
Body mass index (BMI) >30	diabetes, hypertension, joint pains
Unplanned weight loss	medical referral needed
Exercise	lack of exercise can lead to obesity, CHD, diabetes
Smoking	many cancers, respiratory disease, CHD
Alcohol abuse	cirrhosis of liver, accidents at work and on road, hypertension
Glycosuria	diabetes, impaired glucose tolerance
Proteinuria	renal disease, urine infection
Haematuria	prostate disease, urine infection, bladder disease
Travel (for leisure or work)	sexually transmitted infections, food hygiene, malaria, infectious diseases, accidents, skin cancer
Current chronic disease	compliance

---

for specialist advice. Brief interventions to encourage men to moderate their alcohol intake can be beneficial (Edwards 2004a).

It is unrealistic to advise on all the above issues in one short consultation. Further support should be offered for any area of concern, for example smoking cessation, diet, weight, blood pressure and lipid screen. Any screening process, including well-men checks, can be regarded in both positive and negative terms. Screening may confirm that an individual is in good health now, but it does not guarantee continued health. It could be argued that diagnosing a disease before it manifests with symptoms is beneficial to the patient. Conversely, it may increase stress and anxiety. Men who prefer not to be screened for any condition must have their views respected (see Chapter 1, Respect for autonomy).

Key issues to be included in a holistic consultation can be seen in Box 5.1. This is not intended to be a comprehensive list, but a reminder of the many facets of health that must be assessed.

Improving men's health

Although men have historically been complacent or neglectful of their health, men's health appears to receive a higher profile in 2007 through media reports and journals. Health professionals must be abreast of current developments and discussions if they wish to offer support in the battle to increase knowledge and awareness of men's health issues.

If the risk factors for preventable disease are explained and support for lifestyle modification is offered, the individual will have the knowledge with which to make an informed decision about his future lifestyle. Inevitably some men will continue to follow an unhealthy lifestyle. This is their choice and must be respected, despite Government pressure to change peoples' lifestyles.

Never make assumptions about men and their attitudes to health but be proactive in offering health advice and support.

Activity 5.2

Carry out an analysis job to identify all men over 40 years of age who do not have a record of a blood pressure reading in the past three years. Invite them for a well-man check. Audit the findings.

The next section aims to provide the reader with an insight into the complexity of issues surrounding the aetiology and screening of testicular and prostate cancers that will enable them to support their male patients.

Testicular cancer

Incidence

Although testicular cancer is still uncommon, cases have increased from just over 1500 new cases a year in the UK (Imperial Cancer Research Fund 1997), to almost 2000 new diagnoses a year (Cancer Research UK 2006). The incidence rate has more than doubled over the mid-1980s and is now the most common cancer among men aged between 15 and 44, although over 9 in 10 patients are cured (Cancer Research UK 2006).

Aetiology

Genetic, hormonal and environmental factors are thought to contribute to the development of testicular cancer (Summers 1995). A testicular cancer gene abnormality called TGCT1 (Testicular Germ Cell Tumour1) has been found on the X chromosome, suggesting it is inherited from the mother. Testicular cancer is more common in Northern Europe and generally rare in nonCaucasian men (Cancer Research UK 2006). Statistics highlight a consistent reduction in black, compared with white, American men, suggesting a genetic component to the disease. However, the rates rise in African and other nonCaucasian migrants to the USA, suggesting the influence of some environmental factor(s) (Rosella 1994).

Testicular cancer is still most common in affluent Caucasians (Cancer Research UK 2006). The young age onset of this cancer, and social mobility of many men during their working lives, has persistently cast doubt on the role of occupation in aetiology.

Although there are no known causes for the rising incidence of testicular cancer, possible factors have been proposed (Box 5.2).

Symptoms

Testicular cancer usually presents as a painless enlargement of one testicle (Box 5.3). The absence of pain initially, combined with a lack of knowledge, often causes men to delay seeking medical advice. Very rarely, the tumour may disappear and the first symptom is backache from metastases.

Diagnosis

The doctor will examine and reassure a man who has a benign lump. Intrascrotal masses in young men can be secondary to non-malignant disease. An ultrasound will suggest a cancerous growth, which is confirmed after biopsy

---

Box 5.2 Suggested risk factors for testicular cancer (ICRF 1997, Moore and Topping 1999, CRUK 2006)

Past medical history of:

- undescended testicles increases the risk by 5–10 fold. If corrected before age six years reduces the risk, but still higher than men without undescended testicles
- inguinal hernia
- testicular torsion
- testicular trauma
- mumps/orchitis
- prenatal exposure to oestrogen

Other factors:

- aged 15–49
- white – testicular cancer is four times more common amongs white than black males
- early age of puberty
- rare familial syndromes
- close family relatives (brother or father) with testicular cancer increases the risk ten-fold
- wearing tight underwear
- central heating
- hot baths

Box 5.3 Symptoms of testicular cancer

In the early stages of the disease the man might notice:

- a painless enlargement of one testicle
- a vague 'heaviness' in the scrotum or groin
- a sore that does not heal

As the disease spreads he may feel:

- a dull ache in the groin or lower abdomen
- backache
- alteration in the firmness of the testes
- a hard, small irregular lump on palpation when the cancer has infiltrated to the lymph nodes or bones

and microscopic examination. In some cases, diagnosis can only be made by surgical exploration. Testicular cancers may be germ cell tumours, seminomas (usually malignant), teratomas (benign tumours) or of mixed aetiology. Teratoma usually affect men aged 15–30 years; seminomas are more common in men aged 30–50 years.

Treatment

Testicular cancer is highly susceptible to modern treatments and the vast majority of men are cured, with an overall survival rate of over 95% (Cancer Research UK 2006), although if treatment is delayed the disease can be fatal.

Normally surgery will be carried out to remove the affected testicle (orchidectomy); cancer of both testicles is rare. Chemotherapy is usually given for metastastic spread, while radiotherapy will successfully treat almost all men with slow growing testicular cancer.

Fertility

The loss of one testicle per se does not affect fertility, although treatment with radiotherapy or chemotherapy can affect fertility for 12–24 months (Imperial Cancer Research Fund 1997). There is no evidence of any genetic risks from treatment in children fathered by men treated for testis cancer.

Altered body image

A man who loses a testicle, for whatever reason, can suffer shame and distress, with a psychological loss of self-esteem (Blackmore 1989). He feels less masculine, less virile and less able to perform sexually, although the latter may be perceived loss of sexual function. The anxiety and depression that follow orchidectomy can last for several years.

Testicular self-awareness

Testicular cancer is still relatively uncommon compared with other cancers, but there is clearly a need for a change in attitude to the role of men in society. Evidence suggests that early detection of testicular cancer improves morbidity and mortality. However, it has been reported that less than 1 in 5 men regularly examine their testicles (McCullagh, Lewis & Warlow 2005). Sanden, Larsson & Eriksson (2000) reported that few men had any explicit prior knowledge of testicular cancer before their tumours were detected.

Men need to take an active part in health promotion and disease prevention, be aware of changes in their body and to visit a doctor in time; none of
the 21 men interviewed post-operatively for testicular cancer routinely
inspected his body (Sanden et al. 2000).

Results of a descriptive survey of 203 students indicated that the majority
of respondents were either uninformed or misinformed about the risks and
symptoms of testicular cancer, although 78% indicated an interest in accessing information (Moore & Topping 1999). Men need a clearer understanding
of the role of testicular self-examination (TSE) and its importance in reducing
morbidity and mortality through early detection.

TSE is a simple, effective screening procedure that is easily taught and
practised. Tugwell (1996) demonstrated the benefits of teaching TSE in her
audit of military personnel, although a minority of men thought that this
topic should not be discussed. There is no normal testicular size or shape;
all men from the onset of puberty should be aware of what is normal for
them. This parallels the advice given to women for breast awareness. TSE
should be carried out routinely, and is most easily done after a warm bath
or shower when the scrotal sac is relaxed. The testes should feel firm and
smooth. Any change or irregularity should be discussed with a doctor. Reassure men that the majority of lumps are benign.

TSE is as controversial as breast self-examination. Morris (1996) argued
that TSE raises undue anxiety, inevitable false positives, and increased
GP consultations and hospital referrals. These are all pertinent issues for
any screening process, which have not prevented women's health screening to progress, and should not prevent promotion of men's health
screening.

Nurses must feel comfortable, and not embarrassed, to discuss this procedure with young men. It is inevitable that some young men will be embarrassed by any mention of their genitalia, but a professional approach by the
nurse can defuse this embarrassment.

Literature that reinforces the information can be read at leisure and shared
with friends and family. TSE leaflets should be readily available for men and
women (wives, mothers, girlfriends, partners) in the surgery. It has been
suggested that men can identify with photographic visual aids, which are
more realistic than diagrammatic aids, although the sensitivity of cultural
issues must not be ignored (Peate 1997).

Testicular awareness should be included in all health promotion/well-
men health checks, particularly for men under 49 years (Box 5.4). However,
over-palpation of the testes may result in `self-palpation orchitis', which can
mimic referred pain (Holland, Feldman & Gilbert 1994), so sensible advice
should be given.

Box 5.4   Role of the nurse in testicular self-awareness

- Raise the subject as part of a health check
- Determine level of awareness of testicular disease
- Ask about past medical/family history – is there a risk factor?
- Discuss TSE if appropriate
- Reinforce with leaflet if required
- Emphasise that most lumps are benign
- Encourage man to seek medical advice if any change in the testes
- Advise on a healthy lifestyle.

Prostate cancer

Three main areas of concern and controversy surrounding prostate cancer are risk, screening and management. Nurses will encounter many men with prostastic symptoms in general practice and will be expected to answer questions relating to tests for, and management of, prostate cancer. When the arguments for and against prostate screening have been examined, the nurse may feel more competent to answer some of these questions.

Incidence (Cancer Research UK 2005)

Cancer of the prostate is the most common cancer in men in the UK, accounting for 1 in 5 of all new male cancers diagnosed, and 13% of male deaths from cancer. In 2001 there were 30,142 new cases of diagnosed prostate cancer in the UK, with a reported lifetime risk of diagnosis of 1 in 13. Few cases are reported in men less than 50 years, with more than 63% of cases in men over 70 years; prostate cancer accounts for 26% of all cancer deaths in men aged 85 and older.

However, many men have a slow growing cancer that does not spread, resulting in men dying with the disease rather than from it, as only 1 in 25 men with the disease will die from it. Survival from prostate cancer is strongly related to the stage of disease at diagnosis. The high mortality rate may be due to the fact that it is often only detected in its advanced stages.

Aetiology

There is no one specific factor that causes prostate cancer. Suggested risk factors are summarised in Box 5.5. Insulin-like growth factor (IGF-1) is a protein involved in normal cell proliferation and death. Cancer Research UK

Box 5.5   Risk factors for prostate cancer (Cancer Research UK 2005)

- Risk increases with age – low risk in men under 50
- More common in black men than white – lowest risk in Far Eastern and Asian men
- Family history of prostate cancer – higher risk if brother affected rather than father
- Family history of breast cancer
- Exposure to cadmium or radiation
- High fat, low green vegetable diet
- Insulin-like growth factor (IGF-1) – requires further investigation.

(2005) reported a meta-analysis that found higher concentrations of IGF-1 were associated with an increased risk of prostate cancer. There is no strong evidence that either smoking or vasectomy is associated with prostate cancer.

Diagnosis

Presenting symptoms that relate to enlargement of the prostate gland usually involve bladder outflow obstruction, resulting in difficulty in passing urine, although in most cases the enlargement is benign. Men who have prostate cancer may also be asymptomatic. Men are advised to seek medical advice if they have difficulty passing urine, get up regularly several times in the night to pass urine or pass blood in their urine. The disease is diagnosed by a urologist only after several investigations.

Prostate-specific antigen

The role of prostate-specific antigen (PSA) is to liquefy semen. It is not normally found in the blood, except in very small amounts when leaked into the bloodstream. A blood test for PSA measures prostate tissue rather than prostate cancer; the PSA can show false positive and false negative results for cancer. Approximately 20% of all identified prostatic lesions are accompanied by a normal serum PSA (Lopez-Saez et al. 2004), while Oliffe (2006) reports that between 67% and 92% of men who have a positive PSA test will not have prostate cancer. Prostatits can lead to a raised PSA. However, up to 1% of men under the age of 50 with a normal PSA will go on to develop invasive cancer in the next 10 years, with a slightly higher preponderance in older men (University of York 1997). Normal PSA values are shown in Box 5.6.

Box 5.6   Normal and abnormal PSA results

- 0–4 ng/ml – normal for men up to 60 years old
- up to 6.5 ng/ml – normal for men in their 70s
- 6.5–10 ng/ml – there may be a problem with the prostate
- >10 ng/ml – may indicate cancer

Digital rectal examination

On rectal examination a prostate cancer may feel enlarged, hard and fixed. This is not an accurate assessment when taken in isolation. Digital rectal examination (DRE) is reported to have limited effectiveness in detecting anterior to midline lesions and small lesion prostate cancers (Oliffe 2006).

Transrectal ultrasound (TRUS) and biopsy

TRUS is performed via a rectal probe, and is reported to reveal potentially malignant prostate lesions while they are still small (Lopez-Saez et al. 2004). A needle biopsy may be taken during this procedure to assess the grade and type of cancer. Complications of needle biopsy include infection and blood may be noticed in the faeces, urine or semen. Even with antibiotics, there is a risk of urinary tract infection, so men must be advised to report symptoms or generally feeling unwell with pyrexia following this procedure.

Treatment

There are several treatment options for localised prostatic cancer (Box 5.7).

Box 5.7   Treatment options for prostate cancer

- Watchful waiting (active surveillance) – waiting to see how the disease progresses before choosing an invasive treatment option
- Partial or radical prostatectomy – to remove malignant cells
- Radiation – may be used to eliminate all cells, or as a palliative measure
- Hormonal therapy – may be used before or after surgery or radiotherapy
- Chemotherapy – usually last resort to improve the quality of life

---

Surgery

The advantages of surgery include the psychological aspect, of something being done, and the option for further treatment if required. There are several recognised disadvantages. Radical prostatectomy can result in incontinence, bowel injury stricture and impotence. Figures for impotency vary. Dearnaley (1993) reported that with skilled surgery, over 95% of men retain continence, while 50% will retain potency. Hanbury and Sethia (1995) reported that 2.9% of men in their study were totally impotent following transurethral prostatectomy, while 17.5% had reduced potency. The risk of impotence was directly related to capsular perforation at the time of surgery. These figures conflict with the University of York (1997) data (Table 5.1). Surgery is generally restricted to younger fit men who have no lymph gland involvement (Dearnaley 1994).

Radical radiotherapy

This may be used if surgery is not an option, for example when the cancer has metastasised. Radiation is also an option as a second-line treatment following surgery. Advantages of radiotherapy include the ability to treat a wide margin of pelvic tissue. Disadvantages include a procedure time of about seven weeks, erectile dysfunction and urinary and bowel problems (Payne 2006). New technology means that high dose radiotherapy can be given directly into the prostate via needles (Payne 2006). Radiotherapy is also used for the palliative management of bone metastases.

Watchful waiting (Active Surveillance)

Watchful waiting (or *Active Surveillance*) is precisely what is says; monitoring of the PSA and symptoms to assess progress of the disease. This may involve regular scans and biopsies. Active treatment is undertaken if the PSA levels rise or symptoms worsen. The aim is to delay surgery for as long as possible, recognising the consequences of surgery on the man's future quality of life. It has been suggested that men may be pushed into more invasive treatments by friends and family (Kronenwetter et al. 2005).

Table 5.1 Outcome following surgery and radiation for every 1000 men with prostate cancer (University of York 1997)

Outcome	Treated with surgery	Treated with radiation
Die due to treatment	3–20	2–5
Experience impotence	200–850	400–670
Develop urinary incontinence	10–850	10–30

Hormonal treatment (Anti-androgens)

Most prostatic cancers regress when treated by the conventional first-line approach to androgen withdrawal, although the remission is temporary (Muir & Stratton 1993). Cancers that shrink in response to male hormone deprivation will subsequently recur in a mean of 15–18 months later. Hormonal therapy may be given for 3–4 months prior to radiotherapy and for two years after. This will depend on the grade of cancer and the patients' experience of the treatment (Payne 2006).

While all hormone treatment causes loss of libido, erectile dysfunction and weight gain, tablet therapy also causes gynaecomastasia (growing breasts). The man may then undergo mastectomy. The reader is referred to the British National Formulary for details of the range of current therapies and side effects. The nurse must be aware of these in order to support men undergoing treatment.

Screening

Screening identifies diseases in an asymptomatic person and is controversial, mainly due to the financial cost to the NHS versus extended life expectancy and increased anxiety to the patient. PSA estimation is said to improve the detection of prostate cancer confined to the gland by as much as 78% over DRE (Schroder 1995). Tandem use of DRE and PSA testing for primary screening has proved to be effective, although there is a need for clear explanation of treatment options at diagnosis of cancer (Howe 1994).

The benefits of breast cancer screening are said not to apply to prostate cancer (University of York 1997), but PSA testing to detect prostate cancer will be made available, supported by information about the risks and benefits, to empower men to make their own choice (Department of Health 2000b). To date there has been no publicity about this venture.

What do the men want?

Some men choose not to be screened when fully informed about the risks and benefits of prostate screening (Handley & Stuart 1994), although Howe (1994) suggests that a majority of patients will choose surgery or radiation in the hope of achieving a cure despite the risks of significant side-effects.

It has been reported that many men want to know if they have a disease, even if there is no proven treatment (Woolf 1994). In a 1997 Gallup survey, 92% of men across all age groups said they would go for prostate screening if it were easily available, once they were aware that earlier detection would help prevent future kidney problems (Men's Health Matters/Gallup 1997).

Early detection and prompt treatment may improve functioning and quality of life, even if it does not extend life; conversely it may produce many side effects including pain and anxiety about outcomes (McGovern et al. 2004).

Prostate cancers are not predictable, and vary from slow growing to aggressive and lethal tumours. No screening or management method will suit all men.

Supporting men in practice

Some men, and their families, will have obtained a mass of information from friends, colleagues, the Internet, helplines, and may suffer information overload, which will be confusing. Information and support required will vary for each patient. A realistic role for the nurse includes (Edwards 2004b):

- asking questions about urinary symptoms during well-men consultations
- referring men to the GP for examination when appropriate
- discussing and offering information on prostate health
- encouraging a reduction in dietary fats
- increasing omega 3 fish oils
- advising on dietary anti-oxidants, which may help in the prevention of prostate cancer – these include lycopenes (found in tomato products), Vitamin E and selenium (Dunsmuir 2006)
- dispelling myths about prostate cancer
- provide support to men pre and post screening, and for men diagnosed with the disease
- administering hormonal injections – this offers an opportunity to offer the support discussed above
- considering the family in the patient journey – they will also need psychological support and information.

The nurse may be expected to undertake any or all of the above roles depending on their individual competence.

Activity 5.3

Can you locate information on TSE and prostate screening to share with your patients? Remember women are also interested in men's health. Refer to the useful addresses section at the end of this chapter for relevant websites.

Men who have sex with men

Men who have sex with men (MSM) are first and foremost male, and so are subject to all the other health problems shared by men in general; the general impression is that the only health problem faced by MSM is sexual health (Hart & Flowers 2001). However, certain issues that affect this group must be understood if their health needs are to be met in a way conducive to effective healthcare and health promotion. Key issues will be discussed in the following text. A reader who wishes to expand this knowledge is encouraged to contact gay support groups, attend sexual health clinics in their local area and read more widely about men's health.

Defining the patient group

The choice of terminology used to identify the patient group can be varied. The most accurate definition of this patient group, which includes both homosexual and bisexual men, would be 'men who have sex with men' (MSM).

Some men who engage in sex with other men continue to regard themselves as heterosexual. These are usually married men who are constantly striving to suppress their homosexual feelings, but still engage in homosexual acts in order to satisfy their sexual needs; they end up living what is effectively a double life that can often be full of guilt and stress related health problems.

The population

The gay population, just like any other, comprises men in all shapes and sizes from all backgrounds and social classes. A sizeable percentage of MSM choose to move to the larger cities where there is often less prejudice and a better gay scene, with cafes, pubs and nightclubs. Others may choose, or have no option but to live in smaller cities, towns or villages that have no gay scene at all.

It must be acknowledged that many MSM will face prejudice, violence and rejection from others if they declare their sexuality, so it should not appear strange that they find it difficult to share this information with strangers, as well as friends and family.

Although there is very limited substantial research into the numbers of MSM in the UK, it is generally believed that one in every 10 men has sex with men at some stage in his life. This includes any kind of sexual activity between two men (Box 5.8).

Box 5.8   Sexual activity between two men includes:

- men who regularly have sex with different men
- men who are in long-term monogamous relationships with other men
- married men, who may also be parents, who may have occasional or regular sex with men
- men who have had isolated sexual experiences with other men, e.g. at school or university.

A brief look at the differing lifestyles of MSM will put their health needs into perspective.

Poverty

There is a myth that all MSM have high disposable incomes, good housing and employment. This is far from the truth. Although some may have larger disposable incomes than a family man, within the gay community there are many men and boys who live under very difficult circumstances, particularly men who have been rejected by their family and friends because of their sexuality. The adverse effects of poverty on health are well documented.

Male prostitution

Some young boys end up working as rent boys, or male prostitutes who sell sex to men. Rent boys are as vulnerable to exploitation, sexually transmitted infections and rape as female prostitutes and where there are female prostitutes there will often also be male prostitutes. Because of the prejudice they experience, male prostitutes are far less likely than female prostitutes to report abuse, assault and rape and less likely to seek medical help.

Other health risks

The gay scene itself may contribute to ill health, as much of the socialising is done in bars and clubs (Hart & Flowers 2001). The excessive use of recreational drugs, alcohol and cigarettes are commonplace within the gay club culture for some men. Smoking rates are higher for MSM compared with men in the general population (Greenwood et al. 2005). This may decrease as a result of the public smoking ban that came into force in July 2007.

Many MSM train and tone their bodies in the quest for the perfect body that resembles the bronzed gods constantly seen in media advertising, and which are believed to attract and satisfy partners. Although beneficial to health, there is often illicit use of anabolic steroids in weight training and body building, and excessive use of sun beds, the use of which bring associated health risks. Body image problems and eating disorders are reportedly more common in gay men than straight (Hart & Flowers 2001).

An American study highlighted the continuing harassment of MSM, with younger men more likely to report these experiences than older men (Huebner, Rebchook & Kegeles 2004). Paul et al. (2002) examined lifetime prevalence of suicide attempts of MSM and concluded that MSM have a higher risk of attempted suicide, with a greater risk before the age of 25 years, with risk factors related to being gay or bisexual in a hostile environment.

Older gay men can often find themselves isolated. Some groups within the gay community are very insular and reject men who do not fit into their set.

Bereavement

Men who lose a partner through death or separation need the same bereavement counselling and support services as heterosexual men and women, but may find these difficult to access.

Vulnerability

Not all MSM, particularly married men, are able to or choose to go to gay pubs and clubs to meet people. They may choose to look for sex partners in places that can leave them vulnerable and in danger, such as 'cottages' (public toilets), cruising areas (parks, car parks, supermarket), gyms and saunas.

Approximately 20% of MSM in London are reported to have sex with more than 30 different men every year; half of those have sex with as many as 100 different men, while 10% have sex with up to 200 or more (MetroM8 2006). The physical and emotional health risks of these encounters are vast.

Having so far painted a bleak picture of gay life, it must be remembered that many MSM live very ordinary, happy and healthy lifestyles with the support of caring family and friends.

Adolescence

Clause 117 of the *Learning and Skills Bill 2000* (Department of Education 2000) updated and amended previous legislation, allowing all aspects of sexuality to be discussed in mainstream education. Although not all schools will discuss these issues, it is hoped that there are fewer young gay men left in ignorance about where and how to get help in coming to terms with their sexuality, and how to live their lives in a healthy and safe way.

Coming out

Coming out is being open about one's sexuality. This takes on different meanings for different people. One person may be out to family and friends, while another person is out to everyone. It is therefore important to clarify what the person using the term understands it to mean and in what context he is using it.

It can be a difficult, frightening, challenging and also exciting and stimulating experience. Although liberating, there is also an awareness of the danger of disclosure. There is immense fear of rejection and the loss of all that is important to self and family. It is very difficult for both young and older men to know where to go for help in coming to terms with their sexuality. MSM regularly discuss their experiences, and differences, of coming out. Those who have not been able to come out to their family end up living a life distant from their family. Unfortunately, some men who are able to pluck up the courage to come out also end up living a life distant from their families following rejection.

There are limited positive images of MSM, especially for those who live in small towns. It may seem to the world that everywhere you look there are images of gay life – adverts on television for gay chat lines, gay men and gay lifestyles being portrayed in weekly soap programmes, and gay politicians living openly gay lives. However, life is still very different and so far removed from reality when a man has to tell his parents, siblings, aunts and uncles that he is not what they were expecting him to be. He is unable to fulfil the hopes and dreams they had for him to produce grandchildren and carry on the family name for generations to come.

It is understandably difficult for parents to understand and accept that their son is gay, although surely the most important issue for a parent is that their child is happy in life whatever their destiny. The parents of gay children may find it difficult to locate a sensitive person with whom they can discuss the problem of coming to terms with their son's sexuality. There are support groups in some of the larger cities, although these are not widespread.

It is still common for men who feel that they may be gay, but are unable to come to terms with their sexuality, to get married and have families before they are able to finally accept their own sexuality and find the strength to come out to themselves and possibly, at some stage, to their partners.

Male rape

Very few people are prepared or able to acknowledge that male rape takes place. Male rape is interpreted as a man being forced to have sex with a woman and is treated as something of a joke; something to be desired by 'real men'. Nothing could be further than the truth.

Male rape, in this context, relates to men who are raped by other men. This may be anal penetration, violation or abuse of an individual in a sexual manner. Without doubt a male rape victim will suffer considerable physical and emotional trauma. There is also the risk of contracting sexually transmitted infections (STIs). Few cases are reported to the police because the victim feels ashamed and may, sometimes, wrongly believe that he has been responsible for the attack.

Men experience emotions similar to those of women following rape and may be reluctant to report the incident to the police for several reasons. They may have been cruising when attacked or they may not be out. It may occur as non-consensual sex at a party. Reported cases invariably make it into the tabloid press.

Male rape is not unique to MSM. Straight men are also attacked. The perpetrator of the crime does not necessarily go out to look for a gay man. Men who have been in prison may have been subjected to rape and/or gang rape, in which more than one person is involved in the abuse. This can also occur in sex rituals that some men experience as part of brutal initiation ceremonies into the military services.

A male rape victim may have nowhere to turn for help. The specialist counselling services and telephone helplines which are so valuable to the female victim do not exist for male victims. Limited understanding and support is available from some police forces due to ignorance and prejudice.

HIV, AIDS and hepatitis

HIV and AIDS were launched into the public arena in a blaze of media attention in early 1981. The positive response by the gay community to what is considered by many to have been the most successful public health campaign ever undertaken by the government appears to have lost its impetus. After an initial instant increase in the use of condoms and the practice of safe and safer sex the number of cases of HIV diagnosed among MSM has been increasing since 1999. There were 7275 new diagnoses in 2004, although it is estimated that 34% of people living with HIV are unaware of their condition (Terence Higgins Trust 2006). In 2004, 30% of new HIV diagnoses were among MSM.

Unfortunately there is now an increase in the numbers of HIV positive younger gay males who, when questioned, say that they see HIV and AIDS as a disease that affects older gay men – those in their mid-30s and older. However, it is young men aged 25–39 years who are the most likely to be diagnosed with HIV (Terence Higgins Trust 2006).

Health professionals, in their roles as health educators, must continue to provide appropriate information about HIV and AIDS to all men, regardless of their sexuality as the majority of people diagnosed with HIV in 2004 (59%) had been infected through heterosexual sex, many of African origin (Terence Higgins Trust 2006).

Although it is less publicised, MSM have an increased risk of contracting hepatitis B through body fluids. Hepatitis B is more infectious and more easily transmitted than HIV. MSM should therefore be offered vaccination against hepatitis B as well as advice on safe sex, to reduce the spread of all sexually transmitted infections.

Confidentiality

Research indicates that MSM would prefer to disclose their sexual orientation to healthcare professionals, but are reluctant to do so for fear of discrimination (Stonewall 2006). Confidentiality is integral to all aspects of healthcare and must not be breached (Chapter 1).

Health promotion

The health promotion role of the practice nurse offers the opportunity to provide appropriate information about STIs, with information appropriate to all clients, regardless of sexual orientation.

Information relating to adolescence and sex education, for example on being gay, coming out, safe and safer sex, should be included. Posters and leaflets need to be displayed with other health promotion literature so patients can pick them up unobtrusively. The knowledge that someone can see what is selected may deter some people from choosing leaflets. It is possible to measure the demand for certain literature by displaying a numbered amount.

Posters should depict positive images of gay life, rather than refer to HIV and AIDS. Additional posters and leaflets in the nurses' and doctors' rooms may be more accessible to some patients. An excellent example of a forward-thinking surgery is THE DOCS surgery in the heart of Manchester's gay quarter, which recognised that 25% of its clients were gay. The surgery met the needs of both the gay and straight patients by creating an environment acceptable to all the clients. Posters, leaflets and comprehensive information displays addressed health issues for their clients. Information on post-rape counselling and support included both male and female rape.

Gay patients who are in a relationship can register as a family and are recognised as such. The team have clearly been able to gain the confidence of their patients, who feel the surgery is a safe environment, one in which confidentiality will not be breached.

Domestic violence is an area that also affects MSM, but will be addressed in Chapter 6.

Training

Training needs for staff should be assessed, and specific needs identified. These may include developing counselling skills for post-male rape, those suffering bereavement and the parents of MSM. As noted, suicide risks are high in this client group, and should be considered within the mental health remit. If these services are provided by other agencies, a support and referral network can be developed. Staff should be aware of local support groups.

Local groups

For more comprehensive information and a greater insight, local HIV and AIDS groups and support groups for MSM and their families can be contacted – see the list of useful addresses at the end of this chapter. Some of these groups will be willing to come to the surgery or let nurses visit the group to develop a knowledge base. Posters and leaflets will also be available from these groups.

The role of the practice nurse

As previously mentioned, the health needs of MSM do not differ greatly from those of heterosexual men, except in the key areas discussed briefly above. MSM are often more receptive to health promotion than straight men. If there are 2000 adult males in a practice population, 200 will at some time have sex with another man. The nurse should not aim to be able to identify or encourage a gay client to disclose his sexuality, but to create an environment in which the man will be comfortable to attend for help and support for all aspects of physical and/or mental health related to his sexuality (Box 5.9). Health profiling (Chapter 4) may identify specific needs of this client group.

Box 5.9   Role of the practice nurse

- To create a non-judgmental surgery environment
- To develop an action plan for the primary healthcare team
- As a health educator on all aspects of a healthy lifestyle
- Act as a resource for information about support groups
- To liaise with the health promotion department
- To liaise with local groups
- To develop a resource folder of contacts and addresses
- To refer to mental health services where appropriate.

Activity 5.4

Ensure that the health promotion literature available in the practice includes information on all health issues pertinent to MSM, and is easily accessible.

Summary

There is no doubt that healthcare workers must increase their efforts to target men's health in an attempt to reduce the health inequalities between both the sexes and the social classes, and to reduce morbidity and premature mortality caused by preventable diseases. A flexible healthcare system that recognises the constraints of some male occupations and permits men to talk openly about health issues will be a step towards empowering men to take more control of their health.

The increasing number and variety of health-related articles that are published in the daily/weekend newspapers will inevitably send men scuttling to the doctor or nurse for reassurance or information about different diseases, including testicular and prostate disease. Men may appreciate information leaflets, videos and support while they await their appointment and during their watchful waiting or treatment period. It is important to create an environment in which all men, regardless of their sexuality, are welcomed, well cared for and respected.

Key points

- Men do respond to structured healthcare counselling
- Primary health prevention is the first step towards reducing morbidity and premature mortality from preventable disease

- Nurses must be informed in order to educate
- It is often necessary to seek appropriate and effective information and support for MSM from sources outside the NHS.

Recommended reading

Davidson N & Lloyd T (2001) *Promoting Men's Health. A Guide for Practitioners.* London: Bailliere Tindall.

References

Armstrong D (1994) *An Outline of Sociology as Applied to Medicine 4th edn.* Oxford: Butterworth Heineman.

Blackmore C (1989) Altered images. *Nursing Times* 85(12), 36–39.

Bone MR, Bebbington AC, Jagger C, Morgan K, Nicholaas G (1995) *Health Expectancy and its Uses.* London: HMSO

British Heart Foundation (2006) *Coronary Heart Disease Statistics.* www.heartststats. org (accessed 19 May 2006).

Cancer Research UK (2005) *Prostate Cancer.* www.info.canceresearchuk.org/ cancerstats/prostate (accessed 20 May 2005).

Cancer Research UK (2006) *Testicular Cancer at a Glance.*
 www.info.canceresearchuk.org/cancerandresearch (accessed 30 May 2006).

Cornwall A & Lindisfarne N (1994) *Dislocating Masculinity. Comparative Ethnographies.* London: Routledge.

Dearnaley DP (1993) Clinical overview. *The Lancet* 342, 904–905.

Dearnaley DP (1994) Cancer of the prostate. *British Medical Journal* 308, 780–784.

Department of Education (2000) *The Learning and Skills Bill 2000.* London: HMSO.

Department of Health (1996) *Health-related Behaviour: An Epidemiological Overview.* London: HMSO.

Department of Health (1999) *Quality and Performance in the NHS: Performance Assessment Framework.* London: The Stationary Office.

Department of Health (2000a) *Coronary Heart Disease: National Service Framework for Coronary Heart Disease – modern standards and service models.* London: The Stationery Office.

Department of Health (2000b) *The Cancer Plan.* London: DoH.

Department of Health (2001) *National Service Framework for Diabetes.* www.dh.gov.uk (accessed 19 May 2006).

Department of Health (2003) *Statistics on Smoking Cessation Services in England, April to September 2002.* www.dh.gov.uk/PublicationsAndStatistics/pressReleases (accessed 19 May 2006).

Department of Health (2007) *Gender Equity Audit Project.* London: Department of Health www.dh.gov.uk (accessed 12 September 2007).

Dunsmuir B (2006) *Causes, diagnosis and staging – Prostate Cancer, BPH, Prostatitis.* The ABC of Prostate Disease Study Day. 4th October 2006. Birmingham.

Edgar M (1992) Collaboration between a district health authority and a family health services authority: structured health counselling within general practices. In *Beating Heart Disease in the 1990s.* London: Health Education Authority.

Edwards M (2004a) Brief Interventions in reducing alcohol consumption. *Practice Nurse* 28(5),28, 31–32, 34–35, 37–39.

Edwards (2004b) Prostate Cancer: an Update. *Practice Nurse.* 27(8), 26, 29–32

Family Heart Study Group (1994) Randomised controlled trial evaluating cardiovascular screening and intervention in general practice: principal results of the British Family Heart Study. *British Medical Journal* 308, 313–320.

Fareed A (1994) Equal rights for men. *Nursing Times* 90(5), 26–29.

Greenwood GL, Paul JP, Pollack LM, Binson D, Catania JA, Chang J, Humfleet G, Stall R (2005) Tobacco use and cessation among a household-based sample of US urban men who have sex with men. *American Journal of Public Health* 95(1), 145–151.

Hanbury DC and Sethia KK (1995) Erectile function following transurethral prostatectomy. *British Journal of Urology* 75, 12–13.

Handley MR and Stuart ME (1994) The use of prostate specific antigen for prostate cancer: a managed case perspective. *The Journal of Urology* 152, 1689–1692.

Hart N (1985) *The Sociology of Health and Medicine.* Oxford: The Alden Press.

Hart G, & Flowers P (2001) Gay and Bisexual Men's General Health. In N Davidson & T Lloyd (Eds). *Promoting Men's Health. A Guide for Practitioners.* London: Baillière Tindall/The Royal College of Nursing.

Holland JM, Feldman JL & Gilbert HC (1994) Phantom Orchalgia. *The Journal of Urology* 152, 2291–2293.

Howe RJ (1994) Prostate cancer: a patient's perspective. *The Journal of Urology* 152, 1700–1703.

Huebner DM, Rebchook GM, Kegeles SM (2004) Experiences of harassment, discrimination, and physical violence among young gay and bisexual men. *American Journal of Public Health* 94(7), 1200–1203.

Imperial Cancer Research Fund (1997) *Testicular Cancer Fact Sheet.* London: Imperial Cancer Research Fund.

Kronenwetter C, Weidner G, Pettengill E, Marlin R, Crutchfield L, McCormac P, Raisin C & Ornish D (2005) A qualitative analysis of interviews of men with early stage prostate cancer: The prostate cancer lifestyle trial. *Cancer Nursing* 28(2), 99–107.

Lindholm LH, Ekbom T, Dash C, Eriksson M, Tibblin G & Schersten P (on behalf of the CELL Study Group) (1995) The impact of healthcare advice given in primary care on cardiovascular risks. *British Medical Journal* 310, 1105–1109.

Lloyd T (2001) Men and Health: the context for practice. In N Davidson and T Lloyd (Eds) *Promoting Men's Health. A Guide for Practitioners.* London: Baillière Tindall/ Royal College of Nursing.

Lopez-Saez J-B, Otero M, Senra-Varela A, Ojea A, Martin LJS, Munoz BD & Fuentes JV (2004) Prospective observational study to assess value of prostate cancer diagnostic methods. *Journal of Diagnostic Medical Sonography* 20(6), 383–392.

Matz R (1993) *Men, Masculinity and Male Health.* London: Albany Health Project.

McCullagh J, Lewis G & Warlow C (2005) Promoting awareness and practice of testicular self-examination. *Nursing Standard* 19(51), 41–49.

McGovern P, Gross C, Krueger R, Englehard D, Cordes J & Church T (2004) False-Positive Cancer Screens and Health-related Quality of Life. *Cancer Nursing* 27(5), 347–352.

McMillan I (1995) The life of Riley *Nursing Times* 91(48), 27–28.

Mens Health Matters/Gallup (1997) *Mens Health Matters in the Nineties. Report of the Survey.* London: MHM.

MetroM8 (2006) *Cruising for Sex – Sexual Health for Men who have Lots of Sexual Partners.* www.metromate.org.uk (accessed 12 May 2006).

Moore RA & Topping A (1999) Young men's knowledge of testicular cancer and testicular self-examination: a lost opportunity? *European Journal of Cancer* 8, 137–142.

Morgan M, Calnan M & Manning N (1985) *Sociological Approaches to Health and Medicine.* London: Routledge.

Morris J (1996) The case against TSE. *Nursing Times* 92(33), 41.

Muir G and Stratton M (1993) Mechanism of hormone independence. *The Lancet* 342, 903–904.

National Statistics (2006) *Health Expectancy. Living Longer, More Years in Poor Health.* www.statistics.gov.uk (accessed 19 May 2006).

Nicholson J (1993) *Men and Women. How Different are They.* Oxford: Oxford University Press.

Office for National Statistics (1995) *Health in England 1995: What People Know, What People Think, What People Do.* London: HMSO.

Oliffe J (2006) Being screened for prostate cancer: A simple blood test or a commitment to treatment. *Cancer Nursing.* 29(1), 1–8.

Paul JP, Catania J, Pollack L, Moskowitz J, Canchola J, Mills T, Binson D & Stall R (2002) Suicide attempts among gay and bisexual men: lifetime prevalence and antecedents. *American Journal of Public Health* 92(8), 1338–1345.

Payne H (2006) *Treatment of Early Prostate Cancer.* The ABC of Prostate Disease Study Day. 4th October 2006. Birmingham.

Peate I (1997) Testicular cancer: the importance of effective health education. *British Journal of Nursing* 6(6), 311–316.

Rosella JD (1994) Testicular cancer health. Education on Integrative Review. *Journal of Advanced Nursing* 20, 666–671.

Sanden I, Larsson US & Eriksson C (2000) An interview study of men discovering testicular cancer. *Cancer Nursing* 23(4), 304–309.

Schroder FH (1995) Detection of prostate cancer. *British Medical Journal* 310, 140–141.

Stonewall (2006) *Men and general health needs.* www.stonewall.org.uk/information_bank (accessed 2 September 2006).

Summers E (1995) Vital signs. *Nursing Times* 91(25), 46–47.

Terence Higgins Trust (2006) *Information Resources.* www.tht.org.uk/informationresources (accessed 30 May 2006).

Tettersell M & Luft S (1994) Lifestyle influences on client health. in S Luft & M Smith (Eds) *Nursing in General Practice*. London: Chapman and Hall.

Tolson A (1987) *The Limits of Masculinity*. London: Routledge.

Townsend P, Davidson N & Whitehead M (1992) *Inequalities in Health*. London: Penguin Books.

Tugwell M (1996) Testicular self-examination. *Primary Health Care* 6(5), 18–19, 21.

University of York (1997) *Screening for Prostate Cancer. The Evidence. Effectiveness Matters*. York: NHS Centre for Reviews and Dissemination.

Waller D, Agass M, Mant D, Coulter A, Fuller A & Jones L (1990) Health checks in general practice: another example of inverse care. *British Medical Journal* 300, 1115–1118.

World Cancer Research Fund (2005) *Informed. News on Diet, Lifestyle and Cancer Prevention*. London: WCRF.

Woolf ST (1994) Public health perspective: the health policy implications of screening for prostate cancer. *The Journal of Urology* 152, 1685–1688.

Useful addresses

Cancer Research UK
PO Box 123
Lincoln's Inn Fields
London WC2A 3PX
Tel: supporter services   020 7121 6699
Switchboard: 020 7269 3100
www.cancerresearchuk.org
Research, cancer information, working with the government.

CRUISEAID
1–5 Curtain Road
London EC2A 3JX
Tel: 020 7539 3880
Fax: 020 7539 3890
www.cruiseaid.org.uk
email: officecruiseaid.org.uk

Gay men fighting AIDS (GMFA)
Unit 43 Eurolink Centre
49 Effra Road, London SW2 1BZ
Tel: 020 7738 6872
Email: gmfagmfa.org.uk
Gay men's work: prevention, outreach, support, information, research, advocacy.

The D'Arcy Lainey Foundation (DALAFO)
A nationwide organisation supporting lesbian, gay and bisexual parents, and can advise those who are in the process of coming out.
Tel: 08701 273274
www.dalafo.co.uk

FFLAG (Families and Friends of Lesbians and Gays)
Offers support and advice to lesbian, gay and bisexual people, and their friends and relatives.
Helpline: Tel: 01454 852 418
www.fflag.org.uk

London Lesbian and Gay Switchboard
PO Box 7324
London N1 9QS
Tel: 020 7837 7324
24 hours a day
Lesbian and gay helpline: advice, information, referrals, counselling, publications.

www.malehealth.co.uk
Fast, free health information for men of all ages.

Medical Advisory Service
Patients Communication Campaign
PO Box 3087
London W4 4ZP
www.medicaladvisoryservice.org.uk
General Medical Helpline: 020 8994 9874 (Mon–Fri 1800–2000)
Men's Helpline: 020 8995 4448 (Monday 1900–2100)
Offers information and advice on medical and healthcare matters.

Men's Health Forum
www.menshealthforum.org.uk

MetroM8
London's sexual health directory for gay men
www.metromate.org.uk

Prostate research Campaign UK
10 Northfields Prospect

Putney Bridge Road
London SW18 1PE
Tel: 020 8877 5840
Fax; 020 8877 2607
Email: infoprostate-research.org.uk
www.proate-research.org.uk
Raises awareness, provides information leaflets, and funds research into
prostate cancer.

www.prostatecancer.org.uk
Raises awareness about the disease and political debate about services and
support.
Telephone support helpline: 0845 300 8383 Mon–Fri 1000–1600, plus Wed
1900–2100

Save Our Sons (SOS)
Shirley Wilcox
Tides Reach
1 Kite Hill
Wooton Bridge
Isle of Wight PO33 4LA
Tel: 01983 882876
Testicular cancer information service giving help and advice over the phone.
Also publicises the need for testicular self-examination. Leaflet with stamped
addressed envelope.

Sexual Dysfunction Association
Windmill Place Business Centre
2–4 Windmill lane
Southall
Middlesex UB2 4 NJ
Helpline: 0870 7743571
www.sda.uk.net
Advice and leaflets on impotence and its treatment.

Terence Higgins Trust
www.tht.org.uk
Has offices and centres across England and Wales.

Chapter 6

Women's Health

Georgina Paget, Gudrun Limbrick and Marilyn Edwards

Women's health often dominates health-related data in nursing texts. This chapter examines three areas of women's health, which are less commonly discussed, and where the practice nurse may have insufficient knowledge to address the topics confidently.

It is estimated that 5–7% of the population are gay, lesbian or bisexual, although exact figures are unknown (Stonewall 2006a). Only a small proportion of women will regard their homosexuality as a problem. The chiefly narrative account of the health needs of the 'invisible minority', describing lesbian experiences of the health services, includes pertinent issues relating to general practice.

Premenstrual syndrome (PMS), which affects many women, is poorly understood and inadequately managed. The resulting aggression can be a potential trigger for domestic abuse, while symptoms of PMS may mask a victim of domestic abuse. Appreciation of the underlying causes of PMS may assist the health professional to offer appropriate advice and support to sufferers.

Although domestic abuse is common and has been acknowledged as a problem by the Department of Health (2005), health professionals need the knowledge and resources to advise women appropriately. Although this section refers to women, the process and management can also be transferred to men.

The invisible minority; health needs of lesbian women

There has been much debate in recent years concerning the healthcare needs of lesbians. However, in health arenas, this focus has shifted dramatically since the subject of female homosexuality was first identified. To understand fully the influences affecting the health of lesbians it is essential to examine the historical context of lesbians within the healthcare system. Indeed it was

The Informed Practice Nurse, Edwards, M. (2008), Chichester: Wiley.

not until the turn of the century that the medical establishment focused their attention on the subject of female homosexuality.

Providing equitable health services demands that provision is culturally appropriate, sensitive and inclusive. Thus the purpose of the first part of this chapter is to demonstrate approaches that health providers may incorporate into their practice, creating safe inclusive healthcare for their lesbian clients.

Accessible, equitable and appropriately sensitive care relies on a deconstruction of the notion of a lesbian as a particular sort of woman who has specific health needs related to her sexuality. Lesbians are as similar as, and as different from, all women, but socially constructed concepts of lesbianism entail common experiences that affect lesbian's use of and treatment by the health services. The health needs of lesbians are reported to be one of the most neglected areas in healthcare (Stonewall 2006b).

Indeed much has been written describing a reliance on the need to construct 'the other', the effect of which is to increasingly validate the lives of dominant groups in society and misconstrue and diminish the lives of those perceived to be different. What we have are women who, as a result of their life experiences, become the 'other'. It is hoped that many of such myths can be dispelled, through exploring the common issues in lesbian life experience.

Historical context

Research into the nature of female homosexuality was rare until the 1920s, before which biomedical science strove to classify and label every human condition, ignoring female homosexuality. Lesbians became the 'invisible women' of the twentieth century. Freud's (1920) publication of a book which included a chapter on women and homosexuality led to a change of focus and a hunt ensued for the characteristics of those who suffered from it and how it could be 'cured' (Haldeman 1994).

The inclusion of homosexuality in the *Diagnostic and Statistical Manual of Psychiatric Disorders* (DSM) created a fraught relationship between lesbians and healthcare providers. Visibility for lesbians relied solely on their sexuality being placed clearly within the sickness paradigm, which led theorists to search for a cause, a treatment and a cure for this phenomenon (Haldeman 1994). It was not until the 1950s when Kinsey published the findings of his survey that female homosexuality was recognised as a natural expression of human sexuality. This alteration in attitudes led ultimately to the removal of homosexuality from the DSM in 1973.

Unfortunately this historical context left a damaging legacy whereby lesbians have been found to fear disclosure, rejection and exposure in

healthcare environments and thus remain silent about their lives, their partners and their health concerns (Hitchcock and Wilson 1992; Stevens 1992).
As a result, health providers are often found to perceive homosexuality as a
problem reflecting the attitudes of some sections of the wider community.

Defining the population

Lesbians are women whose emotional, social and sexual relationships are
primarily with women (Phillips-Angeles et al. 2004). The defining factor in
lesbianism is relationships with women but the nature of these relationships
and whether the individual is having relationships with women exclusively,
varies enormously. Some lesbians may have occasional emotional or sexual
relationships with men, or may have had very significant relationships with
men before coming out. Others, in the same position, may prefer to define
themselves as bisexual.

The variety of relationships is as diverse as that in the heterosexual community. Myths abound – the butch-femme dichotomy, predatory lesbians
picking off heterosexual women – but they have no value as patterns, only
as occasional occurrences that add to the variety of the whole. Same-sex
relationships may have a much greater chance of the egalitarianism we all
strive for.

In discussing the health needs of lesbians it is important to be broadly
inclusive in defining the population. Lesbians are firstly women; women
who are as diverse as the population at large crossing every economic, racial,
religious, age and ethnic boundary (Phillips-Angeles et al. 2004). One
common feature of this group of women is their experience of stigmatisation
and marginalisation, which in turn can lead to diminished access to appropriate healthcare.

Self-disclosure

There are no rules, no guidelines to follow. People can become aware of their
homosexuality at any time. With the realisation invariably comes a painful
internal struggle as people tussle with their feelings and the following social
'norm' that has always been expected of them – that they have expected of
themselves. The struggle often happens entirely alone with little in the way
of role models to follow and no one to whom the individual feels they can
trust sufficiently to open up.

For many, information about sexuality is not accessible. Learning about
sexuality is a minefield of rumours, gossip and misinformation. Loneliness,
depression and related disorders (anorexia nervosa) can ensue. Suicide risk
among young lesbian, gay and bisexual people is thought to be considerably

higher than for heterosexual young people (O'Hanlan 2006). Close family and friends may be aware that something is wrong but have little idea of the nature of the root of the problem; they simply do not want to know.

Concurrent with, or following, self-disclosure of sexuality comes the traumatic task of coming out to other people: peers, colleagues, school friends, family. Coming out may be deliberate – a carefully thought-out process of testing the water – or can happen accidentally as other people begin to pick up on signals the individual is unaware they are giving out.

Coming out is a unique stress. The revelation of a significant part of an individual's make-up is seen by some people as socially unacceptable, by others as downright disgusting. Friends and family are seen as potential enemies to the self, leaving the individual isolated and alone.

Coming out is by no means a one-off event. Once the first crisis of self-disclosure is overcome, a succession of crisis points in an individual's life follows as further people need to be told or find out, and the individual goes through a series of questioning of their own sexuality. Some lead a life failing to disclose their sexuality and significant aspects of their private lives to all but a very few, resulting in constant fear of people finding out.

Whether sexuality should be revealed (or will be revealed accidentally) is a decision that has to be made when accessing services, particularly health related services. The dilemma often leads to the individual avoiding the situation completely. Research by a women's sexual health project (SHADY 1996) discovered that 29% of lesbians and bisexual women had delayed using health services. Poor access of health prevention service is still prevalent (Stonewall 2006b).

Coming out may be the first time an individual faces homophobia. More than likely they will have encountered this from schoolmates, colleagues, friends and family. As individuals they may also have been homophobic themselves as part of their internal struggle for acceptance of themselves.

Facing homophobia is like facing a personal rejection and it can come from those closest to the person. There is a huge spectrum of homophobia and, as everyday stress affects each person differently, so the individual's ability to cope with it varies. From overt verbal or physical abuse to discrimination in the workplace, individuals can be stopped in their stride and prevented from living their lives as they would wish to.

Some individuals may come out fighting, others may withdraw into themselves becoming depressed and isolated. Others may need practical support such as legal advice or re-housing. Once faced with homophobia, individuals are far more likely to avoid other situations in which they have to reveal their homosexuality – including accessing services to help them in their current predicament.

Lesbians are as diverse as any other group of people, from varied backgrounds and with vastly differing life experiences. These differences, coupled with anomalies in terminology, have important implications for service providers. Blanket approaches have limited applicability.

External pressures may impact on relationships. Family disapproval (or family exclusion from knowledge of a relationship), for example, is not unusual. Even in accepting families, there can be problems simply in trying to accommodate a same-sex couple in usual family life. Invariably, although isolating, these external pressures only come to the fore where there exists, or they contribute to, problems in the relationship. A lesbian experiencing domestic violence from her partner, for instance, invariably has no one to talk to – and may not be aware of services available to her to help her through the situation. Domestic violence is discussed later in the chapter.

Individuals may prefer to present as single rather than disclose their sexuality through revealing the gender of their partner (Hitchcock & Wilson 1992). This self-negating act can be extremely demoralising especially before the wider family or in the workplace where conversation often revolves around partners and home life. Stonewall offers support for lesbians who want to 'come out' (see useful addresses at the end of the chapter).

Health needs

The assumption is that current women's healthcare meets the needs of lesbian women. In fact, health services are generally not succeeding in catering for their needs. Equal access necessitates services being sensitive to the needs of all communities (see Chapter 4).

Recent research highlights very worrying trends in the uptake and experiences of healthcare by lesbians. A literature review by Phillips-Angeles et al. (2004), found healthcare providers to be judgemental, nonsupportive and negative when a lesbian's sexual orientation was known. This included the disturbing fact that many lesbians decide to discontinue care because of the negative experiences they encounter after disclosure.

Preventative health and women's health services are provided almost exclusively in the context of obstetric and contraception services (Phillips-Angeles et al. 2004). However, O'Hanlan (2006) cites research that reveals lesbians weigh more, smoke more, undergo more weight cycling, have greater abdominal/visceral adiposity, and thus have a higher risk of heart disease than heterosexual women. It follows that the risk of developing diabetes mellitus is also increased, although this is not substantiated (Thomas 2004). Worryingly, some lesbians may not have access to medical information that may indicate a familial history of illness where family relationships either are strained or have broken down (Rankow 1995).

Research conducted by LesBeWell (1994) reported the following typical responses from lesbians discussing why they prefer not to go to their GP practice:

Their attitudes and language put up barriers for me.
These days I will only go for medical treatment when it becomes very urgent.

Reasons given for being concerned about being a lesbian seeking treatment from a GP practice included concerns about:

- confidentiality, both in terms of their homosexuality being revealed to potential employers seeking medical references, and in terms of their family
- using the same GP practice or living and working in the same community as GP practice staff, where the individual's sexuality may be exposed through gossip or accidental disclosure.

Concerns were also voiced that lesbians would receive second-rate treatment if their sexuality was revealed in the GP practice. The following were typical reasons for not wanting to come out to primary healthcare providers.

I'd be afraid they'd treat me differently.
It would prejudice my treatment.

These beliefs often come from past negative experiences of coming out – to health providers or to others – the fear of which is transferred to the current situation unless very positive indications are given that the same negative experiences will not recur. Primarily, however, the fear of revealing one's sexuality comes from a deep-seated understanding that homophobia is widespread:

They would be shocked and horrified.
Homophobia is prevalent in health services.

The following section draws on the findings of research conducted by the health group Les Be Well; its purpose is to examine some of the difficulties experienced by lesbian patients and to offer suggestions for good practice.

Assumption of heterosexuality

I feel that I can't be completely honest with her. She'll say something overtly heterosexual and I'll go back into the closet full speed.

The assumption of sexuality is pervasive in our society. Lesbians easily detect signals highlighting the safety of their environment, and, although these signs if detected may be both subtle and inadvertent, lesbian patients may assume that the practice has not thought about people being gay and that its attitudes are negative. Many of the standard approaches to clients ask questions that only have heterosexual answers before any attempt is made to establish the patient's sexuality. Assessment forms usually query marital status, leaving little room but for a lesbian patient to denote 'single'. Including lesbian patients means substituting 'partner' as an option, providing the practice nurse with significant and relevant information and thus more meaningful and insightful care (Hitchcock & Wilson 1992).

By indicating this level of openness and inclusiveness, practice nurses are in a prime position to create the safe environment required for good rapport and the disclosure of other significant information necessary for accurate diagnosis and treatment.

We'd lived together for 22 years, and she was still referred to as 'your friend'.

Involving a partner in a person's care is seen as good standard nursing practice. However, for many lesbians this never becomes a reality. Involving a partner in care supports the goal of inclusive nonjudgemental care. A thorough assessment of a patient includes discussion related to the patient's home and work life, support networks and her relationship with her family.

Rushing to the conclusion of heterosexuality should be avoided unless explicitly confirmed and this may be achieved by practice nurses reflecting on and clarifying what may seem to be ambiguous information. 'Can I make a note of you partner's name?' Or 'Do you have a partner? What is his/her name?' Such questions imply that the practice nurse has considered the diverse nature of human relationships and allow an appropriate next of kin to be recorded.

Confidentiality

I wouldn't want such information on my records. My family see the same practice nurse.

Worries about confidentiality are commonplace, yet from a practitioner's perspective they may easily be overlooked. Women need to feel safe and have confidence in their healthcare providers (Phillips-Angeles et al. 2004). Lesbians are reported to want to disclose their sexual orientation to the GP but fear they will be discriminated against (Stonewall 2006b). O'Hanlon (2006) cited an American study where one-third of surveyed lesbians had not told their healthcare provider about their sexual orientation. Many lesbian patients are apprehensive about disclosing personal information that may be recorded in their notes in what may be construed as a pejorative manner.

Sharing of information should be done only with the explicit consent of the patient. Including sexual orientation in medical notes can be done with consent and with a relevance to the nature of the problem. Once a lesbian is 'out' there is little a nurse can do to restore what may be a breach in confidentiality (see Ethics – Chapter 1).

Sexual health

I was told I didn't need smear tests – being gay.

For many women the most likely initial interface with a practice nurse is the periodic smear test. Lesbians may previously have been advised that they do not require cervical smear testing. As a result many women present at longer intervals between smears or fail to attend at all.

Suggested risk factors for cervical screening appear to exclude lesbians from the screening criteria. Yet many lesbians have had earlier heterosexual activity, some are nulliparous, some have increased alcohol intakes and some have delayed child bearing. Robinson (2006) reported that only 64% of 300 surveyed lesbians had had a smear test in the past three years, compared with 80% nationally, yet 69% of respondents had had sex with a man in the past. An American study stated that 75–90% of lesbians reported prior sexual relations (O'Hanlan 2006). All women, whether heterosexually active or not, require periodic cervical and breast screening. The initial encounter with a practice nurse often includes two questions: 'Are you sexually active?' and 'What contraception are you using?' The responses to such questioning may create information that is both incomplete and inaccurate. In a similar way, the use of open-ended questions indicates the value placed on all life experiences. Asking instead 'Do you need contraception?' or 'Are you sexually active with men, women or both?' supports the concept of not making judgements or assumptions about patients (Phillips-Angeles et al. 2004).

Also of concern is the risk of sexually transmitted infections (STI). Transmission of human papillomavirus (a risk factor for cervical cancer), and nearly every STI, has been documented with exclusive lesbian sexual contact (O'Hanlan 2006; Phillips-Angeles et al. 2004).

The lesbian family

Lesbian relationships, like any other, can of course bring great joy, stability and happiness. Children may further add to this joy. There is, however, a need for parents to protect their children from homophobia and non-acceptance of their home lives that they will experience from school friends, teachers, and the extended family. Being 'different' is, in itself, an enormous pressure.

Many lesbians have vehemently defended their rights to create families that do not conform to this rigid perspective. Therefore, many lesbian families include children from past heterosexual relationships, through adoption and fostering, and through artificial insemination by donor. In some cases lesbians may present in a clinic seeking advice on insemination or even child care. Lesbians who have difficulty accessing fertility and artificial insemination services may resort to obtaining unscreened sperm, leaving them susceptible to infections (Bridget, Hodgson, Mullen & Smith 2002; O'Hanlan 2006). They may also miss the opportunity for preconception counselling (see Chapter 4).

Lesbians considering parenting can be advised in much the same way as all women; however, attention to the role of the non-biological parent as an equal parent is essential. Due consideration may be given to the sensitivity of the legal status of lesbian relationships. This may be relevant for consent if the non-biological parent brings a child for immunisation (see Chapter 1, Ethics).

With these changes in family structures a growing body of literature has examined the nature of lesbian families. Some theorists have examined the parenting ability of lesbians, while others have investigated the mental health of children raised by lesbian parents. To summarise, most studies concur that there is little difference between this group and their heterosexual counterparts (Dorsey Green 1987). In some cases, lesbian mothers may actually be more child oriented and motivated. The assumptions made in many custody cases of a weak parenting ability among lesbian mothers clearly cannot be substantiated. Similarly, there is no evidence to suggest that children raised in lesbian families experience greater levels of stress. In contrast many children have been found to be more creative, more aware of their feelings and more relaxed.

Mental health

> I wouldn't want them to think I was mentally ill.

Studies have attempted to counteract negative images with less stereotypical ones, creating more positive and balanced perspectives. Early studies suggest that far from being bad for one's emotional health, being lesbian can have positive effects on it: in general lesbians were found to be more independent, more resilient, self-sufficient and composed. Other studies found lesbians to be better adjusted in some respects than women generally and often to achieve better job satisfaction (Hopkins 1969; Siegelman 1972).

Some studies have suggested that among some health workers there is an assumption that sexual orientation is automatically linked with mental distress. Lesbians do have unique concerns, which relate to life in a homophobic world but psychological illness is no more common than in the wider population (O'Hanlan 2006). Some women have been victims of homophobic incidents, whether it be rejection from family and friends, verbal or physical attack or a denial of basic rights in housing, custody, or employment (Bradford, Ryan & Rothblum 1994; Savin Williams 1994). Some women may indeed have experienced this in health settings. Sensitivity to these realities is vital if the practice nurse is to develop rapport with their lesbian clients.

Internalised homophobia may also lead to low self-esteem and isolation. Sometimes this higher level of stress can lead some women to self-destructive behaviours such as increased alcohol or drug use. In all age groups, lesbians may present in a health setting with stress related physical health problems. By gentle and careful questioning, the practice nurse may be able to reveal underlying concerns and thus address physical problems appropriately.

The Civil Partnership Act 2005 states that GP practices must use posters showing positive images of both same sex and opposite sex couples in waiting rooms (Robinson 2006). Gay and lesbian symbols, for example the Rainbow Freedom logo, can be displayed which indicate a practice's concern for this particular client group. Links with other agencies, such as voluntary organisations, can be useful.

Education is the key to providing nonhomophobic and nonheterosexist care. Nurses need to be knowledgeable about the needs of lesbian clients. If you feel that you need training on how to provide culturally competent care and how to ask questions about sexual orientation, contact your training facilitator. No training will be provided if a need has not been identified.

Premenstrual syndrome

Premenstrual syndrome (PMS) is an increasingly topical and controversial subject that is also confusing, because, despite attention in medical journals, PMS is still disputed. This section will provide the reader with an insight into the complexity of PMS, a common condition with which women present to both the general practitioner and gynaecologist. The first step in helping women with PMS is for health professionals to recognise the importance of the disorder and to distinguish true PMS from the milder and more common psychological symptoms or even psychiatric disorders. The latter have symptoms unrelated to the ovarian endocrine cycle. Failure to make these two distinctions has led to inappropriate and ineffective treatment (O'Brien 1993).

Although its cause remains either uncertain or multifactoral, PMS includes a wide range of physical, psychological and behavioural symptoms. The following text addresses the issues surrounding PMS to enable nurses to recognise the syndrome and offer appropriate support and management to sufferers.

Definition

PMS has been defined as:

The recurrence of psychological and physical symptoms in the luteal phase, which remit in the follicular phase of the menstrual cycle. (Hamilton-Fairley, Holloway & Taylor 2003)

A woman can be said to be suffering from PMS if she complains of regularly recurring psychological or somatic symptoms, or both, which occur regularly in the same phase of the menstrual cycle, followed by a symptom-free period of less than seven days (Taylor 1983).

Blake (2003) adds that symptoms should be of sufficient severity to produce social, family or occupational disruption.

Between 20–30% of women have more severe symptoms that are bothersome, but not impairing, and consistent with a diagnosis of premenstrual syndrome (PMS); about 5% are impaired by the symptoms and have a diagnosis of premenstrual dysphoric disorder (PMDD) (Johnson 2006). PMDD is similar to an affective disorder and is classified by the American Psychiatric Society's *Diagnostic Statistical Manual* (DSM IV) (Blake 2003)

Background

Premenstrual symptoms were recognised by the medical profession in 1931. An American gynaecologist, Robert Frank, used the term premenstrual syndrome to describe the problem associated with the normal experiences of menstruation (Andrews 1994). This was possibly because, in the early part of the century, a woman's fertile years were fewer in number, menarche was uncommon before the age of 14 or 15 years and menopause occurred at 35–40 years. Most women spent their intervening years either pregnant or lactating so the menstrual cycle played a less dominant part in their lives (Mascarenas 1990).

A cross-cultural study of menstruation found that the majority of women in all the cultures investigated reported physical discomfort and that negative mood changes were widely experienced (Woods, Taylor, Mitchell & Lentz 1992).

Some courts of law have accepted PMS as a ground for the defence of diminished responsibility in criminal cases (NHS Direct 2006). Dalton (1980) describes how three women were acquitted of their crimes of manslaughter, arson and assault, having pleaded mitigation with diminished responsibility due to premenstrual symptoms. Her extensive description of individual case studies showed that women who sought help complained of multiple symptoms during the 12 days preceding menstruation.

Aetiology

The aetiology of PMS or PMDD is unknown, although nearly all women who ovulate experience some PMS symptoms; for most, these are mild and brief in duration (Johnson 2006). It appears to be more common in women over the age of 30 and is often precipitated by childbirth (Griswold 2004; Kliejnen, Ter Iriet & Knipschild 1990), and genetic factors (Griswold 2004). PMDD appears to be more common in the late 20s and early 30s, and usually persists until the menopause. Risk factors are reported to be a history of postpartum depression, major depressive disorder and possibly calcium deficiency and cigarette smoking (Johnson 2006).

Contributory factors (Blake 2003; Griswold 2004) include:

- allergies
- hormone changes
- endorphin withdrawal
- fluid retention
- hypoglycaemia
- nutritional deficiencies, such as lack of certain vitamins, magnesium and zinc
- deficiency of essential fatty acids
- disturbed function of the central mechanisms regarding the menstrual cycle
- numerous psychological and social theories.

A survey by the Women's Nutritional Advisory Service highlighted the association between increased caffeine intake, cigarette smoking, low exercise levels and increased premenstrual symptoms (Stewart, Stewart & Tooley 1992). Overgrowth of *Candida albicans* and sleep deprivation have also been implicated in PMS (Griswold 2004).

Kleijnen et al. (1990) suggest that elevated levels of oestrogen found in women suffering from PMS may be due to the body's own inability to break down the oestrogen for excretion due to vitamin deficiency. Oestrogen production is also dramatically influenced when body weight falls below or exceeds 20% of ideal body weight (Stewart et al. 1992).

Research showed that premenstrual symptoms often persisted in women on hormone replacement therapy that included progesterone (Hickerton 1994), and in women who had a hysterectomy with conservation of the ovaries, as it appeared to be cyclical progestogen that caused most of the problems, although symptoms were abolished by hysterectomy and bilateral oopherectomy (Henshaw & Smith 1993). Research also showed that women given oestrogen therapy after hysterectomy and oopherectomy did not develop PMS symptoms (O'Brien 1993).

There has been a growing recognition that oestrogen and progesterone directly affect nerve cell functioning and thus have profound influences on behaviour, moods and the processing of sensory information (Sutherland 1990). Ovulation seems to trigger changes that lead to changes in the activity of serotonin in the brain and possibly other neurotransmitters, and these lead to the typical symptoms (Griswold 2004; Johnson 2006). Women with low levels of serotonin may be particularly sensitive to levels of progesterone leading to PMS symptoms (NHS Direct 2006).

It has been suggested that PMS may be due to negative attitudes acquired during socialisation. PMS researchers and clinicians acknowledge that the variability of PMS can in fact be attributed to its conceptualisation.

Symptoms

Premenstrual distress describes a variety of symptoms recurring in the same phase of the menstrual cycle. This is usually 2–7 days before menstruation and is relieved by the onset of menses. Predisposing factors include stressful or emotional life events such as bereavement or divorce, or psychiatric disorders (Glynn 1993). Symptoms are reported to increase with each successive pregnancy (Griswold 2004).

Up to 150 separate symptoms have been linked to PMS (Griswold 2004; NHS Direct 2006), with common ones listed in Table 6.1, and systemic changes listed in Table 6.2. Depending on the severity of symptoms, a woman's home, work and social life can be severely affected, and her quality of life reduced. Women tend to report their own unique combination of symptoms, seeking help for psychological symptoms, as these interfere most with relationships in everyday life (Blake 2003). Be aware that some depressive symptoms may be caused by domestic violence, which is discussed in the next section.

The character and intensity of the symptoms may vary from woman to woman, and in different cycles. One woman may only be able to identify

Table 6.1 Premenstrual symptoms (Blake 2003; Moos 1968; NHS Direct 2006; Prodigy 2006)

Physical	
Water retention	weight gain abdominal bloating peripheral oedema
Pain	pelvic pain breast tenderness headache/migraine abdominal pain backache muscle stiffness general aches and pains
General	exacerbation of epilepsy, asthma, migraine, rhinitis, urticaria and skin conditions change in bowel habit/constipation/diarrhoea tinnitus numbness and tingling palpitations fatigue

Psychological	
Concentration	depression emotional instability fatigue clumsiness or poor coordination insomnia irritability decrease/increase in libido memory impairment concentration difficulty prone to accidents confusion difficulty in making decisions agrophobia/claustrophobia suicidal feelings mood swings panic attacks
Behavioural	personality changes, e.g mood swings irritability and restlessness lowered work performance absenteeism from work or school avoidance of social activities loss of efficiency sleep disturbance – more or less sleep food cravings for sweets, carbohydrates and salty foods

Table 6.1 *Continued*

Psychological	
Negative effects	low mood
	depression
	tension
	crying spells
	loneliness
	anxiety
	hostility
Arousal	feeling affectionate
	orderliness
	excitement
	feeling of well-being
	bursts of energy/activity
Autonomic reaction	cold sweats/hot flushes
	feeling dizzy or faint
	nausea or vomiting

Table 6.2 Systemic changes during the menstrual cycle

Item	Character of change
Temperature	Decreases at time of ovulation, then sharp rise to a plateau
Blood pressure	Arterial pressure lower mid-cycle
Respiration	Increased ventilation of lung with decreased arterial carbon dioxide tension in the luteal phase
Weight	Some women gain in premenstrual period
Carbohydrate metabolism	Tolerance to glucose is less (fasting blood sugar is higher) during menstruation
Cholesterol	Total serum cholesterol rises following menstruation
Thyroid	Premenstrual rise in basal metabolic rate during menstruation
Skin	Darkening of skin premenstrually is related to increased sensitivity to ultraviolet light; increased sebaceous gland activity premenstrually; fewer active sweat glands during luteal phase
Breast	Premenstrual hyperaemia and increased breast size

one or two symptoms in a mild form in a particular cycle, while women who experience more severe effects may experience several symptoms. Symptoms vary so widely between individuals and even between cycles for an individual so it is likely that different aetiological factors apply to different women.

Effects of PMS

Severe PMS or PMDD can have adverse effects on relationships at work, affecting work performance or causing absenteeism; on the family, as the woman stresses about the effect her behaviour has on her children and her partner; criminally, as the woman may attempt suicide or commit crime (Blake 2003).

Diagnosis

There is widespread publicity given to PMS by the lay press and the media in recent years, and with easy access to the Internet, women themselves often make the diagnosis of PMS. Women will present at the surgery and say 'I have PMS'. Other physical illness must be excluded before evaluating whether the woman does indeed experience cyclic symptoms. The severity of symptoms must be assessed and related to other disorders such as depression, dysmenorrhoea, an endocrine disturbance or another cause.

However, a woman's past experience with doctors will influence her future decisions on the need for medical advice. In a study of women with menstruation, Scrambler and Scrambler (1985) identified that a third of their sample had consulted their GP due to menstrual distress and discomfort. The remainder of the sample did not seek medical help because they felt disillusioned with their doctors. Many women found that their doctors were unresponsive, unsympathetic and unable to help. Most of the doctors were male, which made seeking help more difficult.

The negative aspect of socialisation may hinder the process and affect diagnosis. Studies have suggested that doctors may record the psychological and emotional problems experienced by many women during the premenstrual phase and dismiss them as psychosomatic (Bernstein and Kane 1981). O'Brien (1993) stated how PMS was dismissed by many doctors because their experiences had been limited to observations of their own cycles or those of their wives or female colleagues.

It is hoped that this scenario would be less common with an increasing number of women doctors in general practice. The woman may present to the practice nurse as an alternative female health professional.

The fulfilment of a patient's expectations and requirements when seeking help for premenstrual symptoms may depend on the effectiveness of communication between health professional and patient.

Diagnosis can be made on the basis of history, as there are no specific laboratory tests to diagnose PMS. If symptoms recur cyclically, and are relieved by the start or cessation of menses, diagnosis can be made if the absence of other pathophysiological and psychological disorders has been determined

(Mascarenas 1990). When making a differential diagnosis, physical and psychological factors frequently produce a similar or identified pattern. Care needs to be exercised when relying on self-reporting of symptoms.

The diagnosis can be confirmed with a prospective diary of symptoms, taken over two menstrual cycles (Figure 6.1). The woman should note whether symptoms are present, the level of severity, and the dates of her menstrual bleeding (Blake 2003; Johnson 2006). Symptoms are noted using a coding system chart preferably at the same time each day in order to identify a PMS pattern of symptoms.

To clarify the diagnosis in difficult cases a formal psychiatric evaluation, including detailed analysis, a structured internal and an objective questionnaire may help to distinguish into which category the woman fits (O'Brien 1987). It may help the reader to discuss a difficult case with a mental health nurse before making a formal referral.

Activity 6.1

You may like to do an informal survey of your female colleagues and friends to identify the number who have unmanaged PMS symptoms. List the most commonly reported symptoms and the most common home management remedies. This may help you identify sufferers and offer 'tried and tested' remedies.

Management

A woman will eventually seek healthcare support as a result of a recent crisis or threat from a significant other; most women seek treatment after putting up with symptoms for ten years or more (Griswold 2004). The woman may have tried home remedies and self-help strategies before presenting to the nurse. Women are reported to feel less isolated if they talk to their partners, friends, family and colleagues (Blake 2003). Women who seek help specifically for PMS tend to be from social groups I and II. The Primary Health Care Team should also be alert to the possibility of PMS or PMDD in women consulting for other reasons, for example, anxiety or depression (Blake 2003).

A woman will often be reassured by someone recognising and acknowledging there is a problem (Hamilton-Fairley et al. 2003). Once PMS is diagnosed, a holistic action plan can be devised. This will include advice on diet, lifestyle and stress awareness, with a realistic expectation for outcome of management. Advise a trial of exercise and calcium supplements while the

Code   Symptom

T   Tension

I   Irritability

D   Depression

A   Anxiety

F   Fatigue

DC   Difficulty in concentration

AC   Abdominal cramps

H   Headache

BA   Backache

MS   Muscle spasm

BT   Breast tenderness

WG   Weight gain

S   Swelling of joints (fingers and ankles)

B   Bloating

AH   Abdominal heaviness

The woman is asked to complete diary using the symptom code

Days of month

Month 1   1 2 3 4 5 6 7 8 9 10 11 12 13 14 15 16 17 etc

Month 2

Figure 6.1   Example of a menstrual diary.

Box 6.1   Medical treatment options for PMS (Johnson 2006, NHS Direct 2006, Prodigy 2006)

1. Cognitive Behaviour Therapy (CBT) may help psychological conditions
2. Vitamin B6 (pyridoxine) – see Box 6.2
3. Evening primrose oil – controversial (against – Johnson 2006, for – Prodigy 2006)
4. Diuretics – reduce levels of fluid in body, can help with breast tenderness and feeling bloated
5. Non-steroidal anti-inflammatory drug scan help painful symptoms
6. Gonadotrophin releasing hormones (Danazol) – prevents ovulation
7. Combined oral contraceptive pill – helps to stabilise hormone levels
8. Low dose oestrogen – may need an intrauterine system (IUS) inserted to protect against uterine cancer
9. Selective Serotonin Reuptake Inhibitors (SSRIs) can help with a number of symptoms
10. Surgery – there is no convincing evidence that oopherectomy or hysterectomy work, but may help some people.

---

symptom diary is being completed, as many women will get adequate relief from these measures (Johnson 2006).

As noted above, PMS has a multiple and complex aetiology, with different women experiencing different symptoms. It therefore seems unlikely that a single treatment regime will prove 100% effective for all.

PMS is still not completely understood, although many treatments have been tried. Box 6.1 illustrates the variety of prescribed drugs that are used to relieve symptoms with varying degrees of popularity and success.

Women with psychological premenstrual changes will benefit from counselling and reassurance and those with non-cyclical psychiatric problems should be helped by early identification of their problems with appropriate referral.

The role of the practice nurse

Patients often want to discuss treatments for PMS that they have read about in magazines, many of which can be obtained without prescription (Box 6.2).

Women may be more willing to seek help from practice nurses than doctors, as most nurses are female. Nurses may identify women with PMS during routine well-women or general health checks, either through

---

Box 6.2   Treatments for PMS, which can be obtained without a prescription (Johnson 2006, NHS Direct 2006, Prodigy 2006)

1. Dietary advice
2. Aerobic exercise programme – may reduce the intensity of premenstrual mood symptoms and may reduce bloating and breast tenderness, and depression and anxiety. 30 minutes of walking 3–4 times a week
3. Vitamin B6 (pyridoxine) – may have benefit, but limit to 100mg/day because of risk of acute reversible peripheral neuropathy
4. Zinc
5. Magnesium supplements – may reduce symptoms of breast tenderness, bloating and weight gain
6. Calcium – supplement with 1200mg in divided doses daily. Reduces most symptoms, including all mood symptoms, breast tenderness, bloating, and pain symptoms.
7. Evening primrose oil – has no significant benefits
8. Yoga
9. Homeopathy
10. Hypnosis
11. Acupuncture
12. Reflexology
13. Aromatherapy
14. Lifestyle changes
15. Analgesics
16. Vitamin E – more evidence is needed. High doses can be harmful
17. Agnus castus fruit extract – contains substances that may affect neurotransmitters, and may help some women

---

appropriate and sensitive questioning, or through observation of change of behaviour.

Careful evaluation of symptoms and psychological status (Figure 6.1) must be assessed before individual treatment programmes are addressed. Those identified as having psychological premenstrual changes may initially require counselling, although most may find some relief in being able to talk to an empathetic listener. Stress management, relaxation, dietary recommendations, alternative therapies and psychotherapy support may help some women cope with their symptoms.

Research by Golub (1992) found that women who experience severe psychological symptoms had a lower self-esteem, experienced more stress in their lives, more angry feelings and had less effective coping skills. This clearly has implications for psychological treatment of women who seek therapy for PMS. Women with mild to moderate symptoms may benefit from simple advice about dietary changes and lifestyle recommendations, such as those listed in Box 6.3. Basic advice should include encouragement to reduce external stress during the premenstrual phase, while regular exercise can help to reduce stress and tension. An added advantage of a dietary and lifestyle approach is that it gives the woman something positive to do and helps give her some control over her problems.

Various interventions shown to have positive results include supplements of vitamin B6, which is reported to be mildly deficient in 15% of the

---

Box 6.3   Dietary and lifestyle recommendations to reduce PMS (Blake 2003; Griswold 2004; Hamilton-Fairley et al. 2003; Johnson 2006; The Site 2006)

1. Reduce intake of sugar and junk foods as high levels increase body fluids. Encourage to eat small portions of carbohydrate-rich food every three hours during luteal stage, to improve mood swings and reduce the risk of hypoglycaemia
2. Reduce salt intake as high levels increase body fluid
3. Reduce intake of caffeine, which contributes to headaches, anxiety and insomnia
4. Calcium – supplement with 1200mg in divided doses daily. Reduces most symptoms, including mood symptoms, breast tenderness, bloating, and pain symptoms
5. Limit intake of animal fats. These produce a fall in circulating oestrogen and lactogenic hormones
6. Advise good quality vegetable oil, margarine, sunflower oil
7. Encourage a diet high in vitamin-rich foods, such as vegetables, salad, fruit, liver, milk and eggs daily
8. Limit use of tobacco and alcohol, as their harmful effects include a decrease in the balance of many vitamins and minerals
9. Take regular aerobic exercise to reduce stress and increase feeling of well-being
10. Increase water intake, to achieve natural diuresis
11. If the breasts are tender, a good fitting sports bra may be helpful
12. Learning relaxation techniques
13. Making time for friends
14. Vitamin B6 can be helpful for some women

population, and which causes depression and fatigue (Masceranas 1990; Stewart et al. 1992).

Stewart et al. (1992) discussed research which speculated that the relationship between oestrogen and B6 involves altered tissue distribution and perhaps enhances the body's need for vitamin B6. They also examined the effects of vitamin combinations. Combining B6 with magnesium and multivitamin has moderate efficacy, while vitamin B6 and zinc apparently influence other aspects of hormone metabolism in PMS sufferers. Women should be encouraged to eat food rich in vitamin B6, which includes liver, eggs and milk.

If no significant improvement is shown after self-administration of the above measures, the woman must be advised to consult the general practitioner. Prescribed medication may be helpful if none of the simpler measures are successful.

Failure to progress in controlling symptoms with any method of treatment after two to three months should prompt careful reassessment, which may include medical referral. The nurse must be a resource to inform women who may have PMS symptoms, reassure them that PMS can be successfully treated through lifestyle changes, drug therapies or a combination of both.

Perseverance by the patient and the nurse is necessary, and there may be a number of different remedies and approaches used before a particular combination is found to be suitable. Treatments may take a while to work fully. However, the dramatic improvement in the quality of life of the sufferer when a solution is found is worth the trouble and time to continue to find a solution that alleviates premenstrual symptoms.

Domestic violence (domestic abuse)

Screening for, and supporting, victims of domestic violence has not been seen as an area of priority in general practice (Edwards 2005), but was recognised as a major public health issue and received a higher profile following government policy (Department of Health 2005). Most media coverage relates to women and children, as 90% of domestic violence cases are committed by men against women (Department of Health 2005), but the following text can be transferred to all groups, not forgetting elder abuse (Jarvis 2004). Using the term domestic abuse recognises the range of potential abuse.

This section aims to encourage nurses to be proactive in identifying the problem, supporting the victim and acting as a sign posting resource.

What is domestic violence?

The Department of Health (2005) defined domestic violence as:

Any incident of threatening behaviour, violence or abuse (psychological, physical, sexual, financial or emotional) between adults who are or have been intimate partners or family members regardless of gender or sexuality'.

This may be occasional or on a regular basis (putchildrenfirst 2004). Examples of abuse are listed in Table 6.3.

How common is it?

Shipway (2006a) cites statistics on partner abuse and violence in the UK. At least 1 in 4 women in the UK experience varying degrees of violent assaults from an intimate partner at some time in their lives. On average, a woman is beaten up 35 times before she seeks help. Although physical violence is often cited, women may also suffer financial and emotional abuse. Approximately 30% of domestic violence starts in pregnancy and 4–9 women in every 100 are abused during their pregnancy and/or after the birth (Department of Health 2005). These figures are underestimates, as they are only the reported cases.

If these figures are transferred to your family, social life and workplace, it becomes apparent that domestic abuse affects someone known to you, either as a victim or perpetrator.

Table 6.3 Examples of domestic abuse

Physical	Shaking	Smacking
	Punching	Kicking
	Starving	Stabbing
	Suffocation	Female genital mutilation
	'Honour violence'	
Sexual	Forced sex	Refusal to practice safe sex
	Preventing breastfeeding	
Psychological	Intimidation	Insulting
	Isolating a woman from friends or family	
	Forced marriage	Threatening to harm children or take them away
Financial	Not letting a woman work	Refusing to give money
	Gambling	Not paying bills
Emotional	Swearing	Undermining confidence
	Making racist comments	Calling her stupid or useless

Adapted from Department of Health 2005.

Domestic abuse in same sex relationships

Accurate prevalence of same gender partner abuse is difficult to determine, due to poor reporting, fear of stigma and their difficulty in labelling their experiences as abuse (Patzel 2005). It is thought that partner abuse is as common and severe among same sex couples as among heterosexual couples, although they are less likely to tell a healthcare practitioner if they do not feel able to discuss their sexual orientation with them (Stonewall 2006c) (see also Chapter 5). Lesbian women do not always find the formal and informal support structures, available to heterosexual women, responsive to their needs (Patzel 2005), but merit the same professional support from the health service.

Cultural issues

Women from minority ethnic backgrounds may experience forced marriages, female genital mutilation and so-called honour violence (Department of Health 2005). Half of women of Asian origin who have self-harmed have experienced domestic abuse (Department of Health 2005). Shipway (2006b) raises the difficulties of intervening in cases of domestic abuse when the victim is from a minority ethnic community. Fear of being ostracised by the community, or hunted by the family, can prevent a woman seeking help or leaving a relationship.

Domestic abuse and children

Domestic abuse is also a child protection issue. Nearly three-quarters of children on the 'at risk' register live in households where domestic violence occurs (Department of Health 2005). This can result in short- or long-term psychological trauma from witnessing abuse. The Department of Health (2005) cite a study of 111 NSPCC cases of child abuse where domestic violence was present in 62% of cases. The reader should refer to local child protection guidelines for further information about children and domestic violence.

Presentation in General Practice

The National Health Service may be the first point of contact for women (Baird & Salmon 2006), with nurses the only healthcare professionals who come into contact with victims of domestic violence (Royal College of Nursing 2004). Victims of abuse may not recognise their situation as domestic abuse. They may fear losing their children if Social Services are involved, or worry that no one will believe them, especially if there are no physical injuries (Department of Health 2005).

Women rarely report domestic abuse directly to their General Practitioner (GP), but are more likely to present with associated problems (see Box 6.4), with depression being the strongest predictor of domestic abuse (Mezey, King & Macclintock 1998).

Some women cannot find words to describe their experiences. Most women will tell their doctor about domestic abuse if directly asked, and often want their doctor to recognise the situation and provide advice and support (Mezey et al. 1998). This scenario could be transferred to the practice

---

Box 6.4   Warning signs of domestic abuse (Department of Health 2005; Itzin 2006; Mezey et al. 1998; www.generalpractice.co.uk 2004)

This is not a comprehensive list. Signs include:

- General poor health
- Poor nutrition
- Eating disorders
- Multiple bruises at various stages of healing, and in unusual places
- Bites
- Cuts
- Burns or stab wounds
- Broken bones
- Anger
- Low self-esteem
- Panic attacks or anxiety
- Depression (affects 48% of victims)
- Self-harm, including attempted suicide (suicide rate of 18%)
- Post-traumatic stress disorder (affects 64% of women)
- Gynaecological complaints
- Alcohol and drug misuse
- Signs of head injury
- Signs of strangulation
- Bleeding from the ears, nose, mouth
- Deafness, when slaps to the side of the head have perforated eardrums
- Social isolation
- Recurrent sexually transmitted infections (if forced to have sex with at-risk people).

Box 6.5   The victim's perspective (Hoff 1990)

Victims are often stereotyped
I think the professional should ask . . . A good professional draws the
person out and makes the person comfortable.
Say 'what happened? You can talk to me.' Be caring.

---

nurse consultation. Would you recognise the signs? Would you be comfortable with the situation? Do you have the information to support and signpost to the appropriate agencies? Box 6.5 offers an insight into the victim's perspective.

Women who may be stereotyped and confronted with prejudice include black and Asian women, lesbians, those with a disability, travellers, sex workers, asylum seekers, those with mental health problems, vulnerable adults, the elderly and those who misuse drugs and alcohol (Department of Health 2005).

Screening

Screening tools are not routinely used in general practice, although they are more common in the United States of America. The majority of both abused and non-abused women in US studies are reported to be in favour of routine screening, as they believe it would assist women in getting help (Jarvis 2004).

Routine enquiry is a systematic process that requires the nurse to routinely ask questions related to domestic abuse (Baird & Salmon 2006).

The Abuse Assessment Screen (AAS) is a validated screening tool, which can be adapted to any health setting (see Figure 6.2). Although British nurses may be uncomfortable asking direct questions, this tool suggests an unthreatening introduction, and can be adapted to each health setting. The patient has the option not to answer if she wishes.

Barriers to screening

Barriers to routinely screening for domestic abuse are listed in Box 6.6. Health professionals may be uncomfortable raising the issue of domestic abuse if they have been, or are currently, victims themselves. They may also lack confidence and knowledge to initiate the topic (Baird & Salmon 2006). Women may not wish to admit to abuse, fearing the stigma of being a victim, and fearing their abuser's response.

Suggested introduction and questions:

Violence (abuse) is very common in today's world, and it can overlap into our homes. Because violence (abuse) affects so many people, I now routinely ask all my patients a few questions about violence (abuse) in their lives.

All couples argue now and again, even the best of couples.

1. When you and your partner argue, are you ever afraid of him/her?

2. When you and your partner verbally argue, do you think he/she tries to emotionally hurt/abuse you?

3. Does your partner try to control you? Where you go? Who you see? How much money you can have?

4. Has your partner (or anyone) ever slapped you, pushed you, hit you, kicked you, or otherwise physically hurt you?

5. Since you have been pregnant (when you were pregnant), has your partner ever bit you, slapped you, pushed you, hit you, kicked you, or otherwise physically hurt you?

6. Has your partner ever forced you into sex when you did not want to participate?

With any *Yes*, say 'Thank you for sharing. Can you tell me more about the last time?'

The Nursing Research Consortium on Violence and Abuse (1988) encourages the reproduction, modification, and/or use of the ASS in routine screening for domestic violence (cited, but not referenced in Jarvis 20004)

Figure 6.2 Abuse assessment Screen (AAS) (from Jarvis 2004).

Box 6.6   Barriers to doctors routinely screening for domestic abuse (www.generalpractice.co.uk 2004)

- Doctors' fears or experiences of exploring this issue of domestic abuse
- Lack of knowledge about community resources
- Fear of offending the woman and jeopardising the doctor–patient relationship
- Lack of time
- Lack of training
- Infrequent patient visits
- Unresponsiveness of patients to questions
- Feeling powerless, not being able to fix the situation.

Barriers to nurses' screening (Humphreys & Campbell 2004)

- Fear of client's response
- Fear of inability to respond to the client's needs
- Lack of basic content in educational programmes about abuse of women.

It is not surprising that doctors lack knowledge about community resources, as these are poorly publicised. The author had difficulty eliciting information and resources from her own PCT, and was passed from one department to another. Eventually she managed to access information leaflets for victims and help-line cards, but no posters to display. Baird and Salmon (2006) discuss the partnership responsibilities for PCTs in influencing health inequalities, including domestic abuse, which will hopefully see a proactive approach to raising awareness of this issue.

Doctors cite lack of time as a barrier; a seven-minute appointment does not lend itself to opening Pandora's box. It would, however, be possible to ask the patient to return for a longer consultation if the situation arose. Although in the USA it is routine for doctors to ask patients about, or screen for, domestic abuse, British guidelines suggest that doctors and others should maintain a high level of awareness and ask if the clinical presentation is suggestive of abuse. A UK survey of 254 Midland GPs found that only 10% had received some training in these issues, suggesting a greater focus on education and training is needed (www.generalpractice.co.uk 2004).

Although infrequent patient visits was a cited barrier, the victim may attend with another family member. This may not be the opportunity to raise the subject if there is a suspicion of domestic violence, as the companion may be the perpetrator or family member of the abuser (Department of Health 2005).

Some patients will be unresponsive to questions, especially if they are in denial of their situation. Listening skills and a good professional/patient rapport may elicit a response in subsequent consultations. Women view doctors' responses as helpful if they listen and are sympathetic, but unhelpful if they are hurried, unsympathetic and prescribe anti-depressants (www.generalpractice.co.uk 2004). The feeling of powerlessness is understandable, given the poor publicity and resources discussed above.

The author asked several women patients about their feelings on being screened for domestic violence, for a seminar on the topic. Ages varied from 17 to mid-50s. Without exception they would answer to direct questioning, and did not feel it would be intrusive. They would answer honestly whether the questioner was male or female. When discussing the seminar with one woman, she offered the information that her first partner was violent. When asked whether she had mentioned this to her GP, she replied negatively – but would have done had she been asked. There is, of course, the possibility that some patients will be offended, but this is a risk to be taken.

Is this a role for the practice nurse?

If doctors are regarded as difficult confidants, nurses can be alternative consultants. They will usually be sympathetic listeners, who have longer appointments than doctors, and would not prescribe medication. However they also need training for this sensitive role (Royal College of Nursing 2004).

The Department of Health appointed a domestic violence advisor in an attempt to ensure all nurses take a more immediate role in offering women the information and support they need (Strachan-Bennett 2006). Nurses can:

- Help create an environment in which women feel comfortable talking about abuse and ask key questions when taking a social history
- Be aware of signs of domestic abuse (Box 6.4)
- Establish whether there are children in the household – liase with the health visitor
- Support women who reveal abuse
- Keep detailed records about a woman's injuries and what she reports
- Pass on relevant information about local support agencies, whether or not the woman discloses abuse.

Information cards with helpline numbers and contacts can offer an opportunity to discuss the issue with all patients. Although not a victim themselves, the patient may have a close friend who is a victim. Support literature should be available in different languages (dependent on your practice population), in easy-to-read format, audiotapes and CDs. A professional interpreter, or advocate from a specialist organisation, may be required.

Nurses applying a holistic approach to care place an emphasis on the whole person, including the physical, emotional and socio-cultural background (Forster, Pannell & Edwards 1999). However, nurses can misinterpret the cues presented by women, which can then impede identification of victims (Humphreys & Campbell 2004).

The practice nurse can develop a personal repertoire of abuse-related questions that are comfortable, natural and culturally sensitive, which may be written, face-to-face or computerised. The practice team can be encouraged to become more aware of domestic violence, undertake training to identify victims, and to have the knowledge to signpost to relevant agencies where appropriate (Box 6.7). The nurse must be nonjudgemental and respect a woman's decision, offering continuing support and understanding. Focus on the woman's safety, and that of her children, if she has any. You may be the woman's first and only contact with the health service.

All aspects of confidentiality apply (Chapter 1), recognising the need to share information when the safety of the woman or children is concerned.

Box 6.7   The primary care nurse role

1. Listen, and acknowledge the patient's distress
2. Establish links with voluntary services, such as victim support schemes. These can provide support, practical assistance, and advice on legal procedures
3. Have a display board with information about domestic abuse – posters, leaflets, small cards with key contact numbers
4. Ask for training to gain the confidence to discuss domestic abuse with patients in a nonthreatening manner
5. Be aware of child protection issues and liaise with the health visitor
6. Signpost the woman to an appropriate agency

Activity 6.2

Compile a resource folder for domestic abuse, including local and national help line numbers, and local refuges. Find out who has an interest in domestic violence in your PCT. Liaise with the child protection team to expand your resources.

Summary

Homophobia and heterosexism are not the fault of individual nurses but the legacy of their socialisation. Health professionals have a responsibility to explore their own biases, and work to eliminate attitudes that prevent the provision of compassionate and inclusive healthcare (Eliason 1992). Failing to address such attitudes may be seen as a breach of the nursing code of ethics in which nurses pledge to provide compassionate nonjudgemental care to all.

The treatment of PMS is most likely to be successful if the sufferer is shown care and understanding. Practice nurses are experienced in promoting healthy lifestyles, so PMS management would appear to be an extension of their current skills. It is, however, essential to recognise when initial home management is ineffective and refer for consideration of other methods of treatment.

Identifying domestic abuse can open a Pandora's box, which people may prefer to stay closed. It is essential that nurses are comfortable raising the subject routinely during consultations. It would be reasonable to incorporate training in domestic abuse with the mandatory annual child protection training requirement, as these issues are so closely related; this may require canvassing the training department at the PCT, or through your employer. It is not an option to plead ignorance about the topic. The Department of Health Handbook can be downloaded from the Internet for nurses who wish to increase their knowledge of this topic (see Useful addresses below).

Key points

- PMS is a recognised medical condition
- PMS symptoms can be reduced by lifestyle changes
- The assumption of heterosexuality must be addressed
- Confidentiality is paramount
- Domestic abuse crosses all ages, sexes, cultures and social groups
- Women want to be asked about abuse.

References

Andrews G (1994) Constructive advice for a poorly understood problem. Treatment and management of PMS. *Professional Nurse* 9(6), 364–379.

Baird K & Salmon D (2006) Identifying domestic abuse against women and children. *Primary Health Care* 16(5), 27–31.

Bernstein B & Kane R (1981) Physicians attitudes towards female patients. *Medical Care* 19(6), 600.

Blake F (2003) Premenstrual Syndrome. In D Waller & A McPherson (Eds). *Women's Health* 5th edn Oxford: Oxford University Press.

Bradford J, Ryan C & Rothblum ED (1994) National Lesbian health Care Survey: Implications for Mental Health Care. *Journal of Consulting and Clinical Psychology* 62(2), 228—242.

Bridget J, Hodgson A, Mullen A, Smith P (2002) *Sexual Health. Calderdale Lesbian and Gay Health Action Plan*. www.lesbianinformationservice.org (accessed 2 September 2006).

Dalton K (1980) Cyclical criminal acts in premenstrual syndrome. *Lancet* 2, 1070–1071.

Department of Health (2005) *Responding to Domestic Abuse: A Handbook for Health Professionals*. www.dh.org.uk/PublicationsAndStatistics (accessed 17 September 2006).

Dorsey Green G (1987) Lesbian mothers: Mental health considerations In FW Bozett (Eds) *Gay and Lesbian Parents*. New York: Praeger.

Edwards M (2005) Raising the subject of domestic violence. *Practice Nurse* 29(2), 26, 28–30.

Eliason M (1992) Cultural diversity in nursing care: The lesbian, gay, or bisexual client. *Journal of Transcultural Nursing* 5(1), 14–20.

Forster D, Pannell D & Edwards M (1999) Health Promotion. In M Edwards M (Ed.) *The Informed Practice Nurse*. London: Whurr.

Freud S (1920) *Beyond the Pleasure Principle*. London: Hogarth Press.

Glynn O (1993) Talk about menstrual problems. *Practice Nurse* 1(14), 889–892.

Golub S (1992) *Periods from Menarche to Menopause*. London: Sage.

Griswold D (2004) Menstruation and related problems and concerns. In QE Youngkin & MS Davis (Eds) *Women's Health. A Primary Care Clinical Guide 3rd edn*. New Jersey: Pearson Education.

Haldeman DC (1994) The Practice and Ethics of Sexual Orientation Conversion Therapy. *Journal of Consulting and Clinical Psychology* 62(2), 221–227.

Hamilton-Fairley D, Holloway D & Taylor G (2003) *Women's Health*. Oxford: B105 Scientific Publishers.

Henshaw C & Smith A (1993) The premenstrual syndrome: an occupational health issue. *Occupational Health Review* 45, 16–18.

Hickerton M (1994) Premenstrual syndrome. *Practice Nursing* 15(18), 18–20.

Hitchcock JM & Wilson HS (1992) Personal risking: Lesbian self disclosure of sexual orientation to professional health care providers. *Nursing Research* 41(3), 178–183.

Hoff LA (1990) *Battered Women as Survivors*. London: Routledge.

Hopkins J (1969) The lesbian personality. *British Journal of Psychiatry* 115, 1433–1436.

Humphreys J & Campbell JC (2004) *Family Violence and Nursing Practice*. Philadelphia, PA: Lippincott Williams & Wilkins.

Itzin C (2006) *Tackling the Health and Mental Health Effects of Domestic Violence*. www.dh.gov.uk/PublicationsAndStatistics (accessed 16 September 2006).

Jarvis C (2004) *Physical Examination and Health Assessment 4th edn*. Philidelphia, PA: Saunders.

Johnson S (2006) Premenstrual syndrome and premenstrual dysphoric disorder (Just in time). *BMJ Learning*. www.bmjlearning.com (accessed 13 September 2006).

Kliejnen J, Ter Iriet G & Knipschild P (1990) Vitamin B6 in the treatment of premenstrual syndrome; a review. *British Journal of Obstetrics and Gynaecology* 97, 847–852.

LesBeWell (1994) *Findings of Research into Lesbian Health in Birmingham*. Unpublished.

Mascarenas K (1990) What is premenstrual syndrome? Help and support for women with premenstrual syndrome. *Professional Nurse* 6(2), 72–75.

Mezey G, King M & Macclintock T (1998) Victims of violence and the GP. *British Journal of General Practice* 48, 906–908.

Moos RH (1968) The development of a menstrual distress questionnaire. *Psychosomatic Medicine* 30, 853–867.

NHS Direct (2006) *Premenstrual Syndrome*. www.nhsdirect.nhs.uk/articles (accessed 31 August 2006).

O'Brien PM (1987) *Premenstrual Syndrome*. London: Blackwell Scientific.

O'Brien PM (1993) Helping women with premenstrual syndrome. *British Medical Journal* 307, 1471–1475.

O'Hanlan KA (2006) Health policy considerations for our sexual minority patients. *The American Journal of Obstetricians and Gynaecologists*. 107(3), 709–714.

Patzel B (2005) Lesbian partner abuse: Differences from heterosexual victims of abuse. A review from the literature. *The Kansas Nurse* 80(9), 7–8.

Phillips-Angeles E, Wolfe P, Myers R, Dawson P, Marrazzo J, Soltner S & Dzieweczynski M (2004) Lesbian health matters: A pap test education campaign nearly thwarted by discrimination. *Health Promotion Practice* 5(3), 314–325.

Prodigy (2006) *The Premenstrual Syndrome*. www.prodigy.nhs.uk/patient_ information (accessed 31 August 2006).

putchildrenfirst (2004) *Domestic Violence*. www.putchildrenfirst.net/DomesticViol (accessed 25 October 2004).

Rankow EJ (1995) Lesbian health issues for the primary health care provider. *Journal of Family Practice* 40(5), 486–492.

Robinson F (2006) NHS needs to tackle gender equality issues. *Practice Nurse* 32(3), 10–11.

Royal College of Nursing (2004) *Domestic Violence Demands Greater Training and Multi-agency Response, Warns Research*. www.rcn.org.uk/news/display (accessed 12 September 2007).

Savin Williams R (1994) Verbal and physical abuse as stressors in the lives of lesbian, gay male and bisexual youths. *Journal of Consulting and Clinical Psychology* 62(2), 261–269.

Scrambler A & Scrambler C (1985) Menstrual symptoms. Attitudes and consulting behaviour. *Journal Social Science and Medicine*. 20(1), 1065–1068.

SHADY (1996) *The sexual health of women who have sex with women in Merseyside and Cheshire*. Specialist Health Promotion Service for South and East Cheshire

Shipway L (2006a) Part 29a: Domestic abuse and violence. *Practice Nurse* 31(5), 59–62.

Shipway L (2006b) Part 29b: Domestic violence and abuse – specific at-risk groups. *Practice Nurse*. 31(6), 56–61.

Siegelman M (1972) Adjustment of homosexual and heterosexual women. *British Journal of Psychiatry* 120, 477–481.

Stevens PE (1992) Lesbian health care research: A review of the literature from 1970–1990. In N Stern (Ed.) *Lesbian Health: What are the issues?* New York: Taylor & Francis.

Stewart AC, Stewart M & Tooley S (1992) Premenstrual syndrom: is there a basis for a holistic approach? *Maternal and Child Health* 17(3), 86–88.

Stonewall (2006a) *How many Lesbian, Gay and Bisexual People are There?* www.stonewall.org.uk/information_bank (accessed 4 September 2006).

Stonewall (2006b) *Women and General Health Needs.* www.stonewall.org.uk/information_bank (accessed 2 September 2006).

Stonewall (2006c) *Domestic Violence and Same Sex Violence.* www.stonewall.org.uk (accessed 2 September 2006).

Strachan-Bennett S (2006) Confronting domestic violence. *Nursing Times* 102(6), 20–21.

Sutherland FN (1990) Psychological aspects of premenstrual tension. *Maternal and Child Health*15(12), 362–363.

Taylor RW (1983) *Premenstrual Syndrome. Proceedings of a Workshop held at the Royal College of Obstetricians and Gynaecologists.* London: Medical News Tribune.

The Site (2006) *Premenstrual Syndrome.* www.thesite.org/healthandwellbeing (accessed 31 August 2006).

Thomas DJ (2004) Health needs of lesbians. In QE Youngkin & MS Davis (Eds) *Women's Health. A Primary Care Clinical Guide 3rd edn.* New Jersey: Pearson Education.

Woods NF, Taylor D, Mitchell ES & Lentz MJ (1992) Premenstrual symptoms and health seeking behaviour. *Western Journal of Nursing Research* 14(4), 418–443.

www.generalpractice.co.uk. (2004) *Domestic Violence* (accessed 11 October 2004).

Useful addresses

The D'Arcy Lainey Foundation (DALAFO)
A nationwide organisation supporting lesbian, gay and bisexual parents, and can advise those who are in the process of coming out.
Tel: 08701 273274
www.dalafo.co.uk

Department of Health
Responding to Domestic Abuse: A Handbook for Health Professionals. London: Department of Health, 2005.
Gateway reference 5802. Product Ref: 267795
Also available at: www.dh.gov.uk/PublicationsAndStatistics/Publications

FFLAG (Families and Friends of Lesbians and Gays)
Offers support and advice to lesbian, gay and bisexual people, and their friends and relatives.

Helpline: Tel: 01454 852 418
www.fflag.org.uk

www.generalpractice.co.uk
Comprehensive information on domestic violence from the British perspective.

LesBeWell
An organisation specialising in lesbian and bisexual women's health.
PO Box 4048

Moseley
Birmingham B13 8DP
National Tel: 020 7251 6580

Lesbian and Gay Switchboard
London Lesbian and Gay Switchboard
PO Box 7324
London N1 9QS
Tel: 020 7837 7324
24 hours a day
Lesbian and gay helpline: advice, information, referrals, counselling, publications.

National Association for Premenstrual Syndrome (NAPS)
7 Swift's Court
High Street
Seal, Kent TN15 0EG
Tel: 01732 760012 (helpline)

Premenstrual Society
PO Box 429
Addlestone
Surrey KT15 1DZ
Tel: 01932 872 560

Refuge
A national charity for women and children who experience domestic violence. Operates a network of safe houses and provides outreach services for women and children. Also have some refuges for women from particular ethnic or cultural backgrounds.

24-hour National Domestic Violence freephone helpline run in partnership between Refuge and Women's Aid.
2-8 Maltravers Street
London WC2R 3EE
Tel: 0808 2000 247 helpline
www.refuge.org.uk

Stonewall
Campaigning charity for lesbian, gay, and bisexual people.
www.stonewall.org.uk

Women's Health
52 Featherstone Street
London EC14 8RT
Tel: 0207251 6580

Victim Support
National Office
Cranmer House
39 Brixton Road
London SW9 6DZ
Tel: 020 7735 9166
Tel: 0845 303 0900 Victim support line
www.victimsupport.org for information on local branches

Women's Aid Federation of England
National domestic violence charity (see website for contacts for Scotland, Wales and Ireland)
Head Office
PO Box 391
Bristol BS99 7WS
Tel: 0117 944 4411 general enquiries only
24-hour helpline: 0808 2000 247 Monday–Friday 0900–2100, Weekends 0900–1900, Bank Holidays 0900–1700
www.womensaid.org.uk

Chapter 7

Health Needs of Young People

Susan Jones, Marilyn Edwards and Wendy Okoye

Young people receive most of their health education through school and/or from parents. They do, however, present in the surgery for support and advice for a variety of health issues, particularly diet and sexual health. A parent may bring a child for dietary advice, expecting the nurse to achieve miracles in altering the child's dietary lifestyle. Many of the parents' expectations are, however, unrealistic. This chapter includes nutritional issues that are related to healthy eating within young peoples' lifestyles. Young people appear to think they are immune to the effects of poor diet and an unhealthy lifestyle. The nurse has an important role in identifying eating disorders, for which guidance on management and referral is offered. Health professionals must use any opportunity to encourage this client group to respect their bodies and reduce their morbidity.

General health of young people is briefly discussed, but as young people will continue to have sex, with or without healthcare support, the implications for this are discussed more fully.

Nutritional issues in young people

Adolescence is a time of both rapid physical growth and hormonal change. On average, a girl's growth spurt occurs between the ages of 10 and 13 and a boy's between 12 and 15. With increasing independence and money of their own, missed meals, snacking, cigarette smoking and alcohol consumption become common habits in teenage years. Peer pressure and self-identity are well known to be powerful influences on young people. This section examines the current nutritional issues pertinent to practice nurses when advising and supporting young people and their parents. Obesity is a major health concern, and is discussed in detail before a general overview of relevant nutritional issues. Eating disorders are addressed as a separate issue later in the chapter. Some references from the first edition are still considered most relevant and are included in the text.

The Informed Practice Nurse, Edwards, M. (2008), Chichester: Wiley.

What is a healthy diet for a young person?

The nationally recognised system for teaching healthy eating is to use the eat well plate showing the main food groups and the proportions of these groups that make up a healthy balanced diet. It is available at www.eatwell. gov.uk. The actual amounts of food required vary according to the individual and are indicated in the average portion sizes shown in Table 7.1. The key message to achieve a healthy diet is to eat three meals daily, choosing foods from the main four groups within the eat well plate, which are bread and cereals, fruit and vegetables, meat, fish and alternatives, and milk and dairy foods.

Using a catchy phrase such as the 3Rs can get across the message that eating three regular meals a day is crucial to achieving a healthy diet.

Young people snack more than other age groups, most snack foods are high in fat and sugar, and many takeaway snack foods are now marketed

Table 7.1   What is an average portion?

Food groups	Suggested daily amounts and types of food
Bread and cereals	6–14 measures One measure = 1 slice bread/2 heaped tablespoons boiled rice or pasta/1 small chapatti/2 egg-size potatoes
Fruit and vegetables	5 or more portions a day 1 portion = 1 piece fresh fruit, for example, an apple or orange/1 medium portion vegetables including salad. Fresh/tinned/frozen/dried are all included to dispel the myth that frozen and tinned vegetables are inferior to fresh vegetables
Meat, fish and alternatives	2–4 measures One measure = 3 medium slices meat/fish 4 tablespoons lentils or dhals Choose low fat meats and low fat cooking methods Choose oily fish, such as mackerel or salmon once a week
Milk and dairy products*	3–5 measures One measure = 1 medium glass milk/1 pot yoghurt
Foods containing fat	1–5 measures One measure = 1 teaspoon butter/margarine/oil/1 packet crisps/1 tablespoon mayonnaise
Foods containing sugar	0–2 measures One measure = 2 biscuits/1small bar chocolate/1 small bag sweets/half slice cake/3 teaspoons sugar

*Increased for young people, as calcium requirements during adolescence are higher.

in supersize portions. These are challenging factors to be addressed when trying to encourage the young person to eat a balanced diet.

Overweight

In 2008, obesity is the greatest public health challenge, as we live in an increasing 'obesogenic' society where making health choices is often difficult. The increase in obesity began in the mid to late 1980s. Practice nurses across the country are now seeing more overweight young people in their surgeries, although they will probably present for other reasons, such as immunisations, minor injuries or asthma reviews.

It is estimated that 25 % of 11–15year olds were overweight in 2004 (Health Survey 2004).

The definition of overweight uses the BMI charts from birth to 23 years available from the Child Growth Foundation (see Useful addresses at the end of the chapter). The adult BMI values used on the computer system within general practice is accurate for people only over the age of 16 years. The equation, weight ÷ height^2, needs to be worked out individually and plotted according to age on the gender appropriate BMI chart. Clinically a BMI over the 91st centile is considered overweight and over the 98th considered obese. However, epidemiological studies use a more stringent definition; that is a BMI over the 85th centile is overweight and over the 95th centile is classed as obese. Referral to an appropriate specialist should be considered for young people who have BMI over the 98th centile and co-morbidity, for example diabetes (National Institute for Clinical Excellence 2006).

Being overweight is due to a balance of more food energy being eaten than being used. In the 1950s the general amount of activity was equivalent to a marathon per week but nowadays it is far less. Approximately 30% of boys and 40% of girls are not participating in one hour a day of physical activity (Department of Health 2004). Young people who have either one or both parents overweight are more likely to be overweight than children with normal weight parents. Other groups that are more predisposed to being overweight are those with learning disabilities, from deprived backgrounds, black and minority ethnic groups and looked after children. The reasons for this are complex, but are associated with less physical activity, more screen (television and computer) viewing and diets low in fruit and vegetables.

Although the causes of being overweight are many, the lifestyle changes required to achieve weight loss are the same for everyone; these are to eat three regular meals and increase daily physical activity. Another issue to consider is the apparent low level of parental awareness of their child's obesity (personal observation); sensitivity is therefore essential to avoid alienating the family. Less diplomatic approaches can result in complaints to the practice and time-consuming consultations to engage with the family.

The effect of being overweight on the young person is associated with low self-esteem, bullying, disordered eating and social isolation. The serious health risks of being overweight have been recognised by Rudolph et al. (2006). These are:

- insulin resistance and type 2 diabetes – acanthosis nigrans is a marker for development of type 2 diabetes (marking on skin of arms, trunk, legs)
- sleep apnoea and asthma
- high blood pressure and subsequent cardiovascular disease as an adult
- orthopaedic complications
- some cancers.

The current evidence for effective interventions for managing childhood obesity is disappointing due to a lack of robust trials. The very best outcome that can be expected is a reduction in BMI of 10%. However, realistically in the author's experience, *weight maintenance* is a great achievement for many of the young people, as escalating weight gain seems all too common. Nationally there are several initiatives to manage overweight young people, including the *Watch It* programme in Leeds (Rudolph et al. 2006). The *MEND* programme (Mind, Exercise, Nutrition and Do-It) originated from Great Ormond Street Hospital, and at the time of writing is being spread nationally through local groups, such as the *Fit Club* in Wolverhampton, with the help of lottery money. The groups meet weekly, involve fun activities and education and are led by a variety of personnel such as youth workers, community workers, dieticians and psychologists.

It is important to be aware that the young person's self-esteem may be low, so the consultation needs to be handled with care to enable the teenager to leave feeling more hopeful. Most of us know what we need to do to lose weight but modern lifestyles put perceived obstacles in the way. The more effective consultation involves the use of open questions, which is more likely to motivate suggestions from the family of small lifestyle changes.

Interestingly there is now evidence from sleep studies and the Avon longitudinal study that good sleep can help with obesity prevention. Commonsense indicates that good sleep can be promoted by removal of television, computers and gadgets from the bedroom (Taheri 2006). This may seem draconian to both adolescents and adults alike!

What can the practice nurse do?

- At the first consultation it is useful to make the interaction as supportive as possible. Emphasise that the whole family needs to be involved in lifestyle changes. It is ineffective if the session is just targeted at the young person.
- Use the plate model as a teaching tool and discuss the choice of a wide variety of meals from the four main food groups with a minimum of foods from the fatty and sugary group. Also use a seven-inch diameter plate to illustrate portion sizes. Often portion sizes for the family need altering to fit smaller plates, with half the plate comprising vegetables/salad and the rest being a small amount of meat, fish or vegetarian option with a portion of carbohydrate from the bread and cereal group.
- Discuss the value of eating three regular meals and very few snacks. The *Watch It* programme uses anagrams such as consider the three Ss. Only eat when **S**itting, **S**ocialising and **S**lowly, which is a fun way of getting the message across. Acknowledge that, to be successful, the young person needs to want to lose weight. They need positive, continual support from family and friends.
- Constant nagging is counterproductive.
- Acknowledge that the widespread advertising and acceptability of snack foods is a hindrance to making changes to achieve weight loss. Discuss tactics to change choices of snack foods, including distraction activities.
- Promote increased habitual physical activity for the whole family, for example, using stairs rather than escalators, taking up cycling, and accessing facilities at local leisure centres.
- Ask open questions with the aim of motivating the family to suggest making small changes to their lifestyle. A maximum of three changes is realistic to begin with. Common changes include buying more fruit in place of biscuits in the home, walking together at weekends, and eating vegetables seven days a week.
- Discuss short-term goals with treats for achieving the agreed targets. These could include a trip out, magazines or fashion jewellery/accessories. Ask open questions to facilitate suggestions for spending pocket money on items other than food (such as saving for bigger items).
- Stress value of adequate sleep and bedtime routine to prevent obesity.
- Inform the family that limiting television and screen watching to less than 2 hours a day is helpful in the effort to increase activity and promote weight loss (Hancox, Milne & Poulton 2004).

- Ask the young person what activities they enjoy doing to demonstrate there is life beyond being overweight.
- Liaise with the local community dietician, health promotion unit and school nurses for further information. They may have run suitable groups.
- If the family agrees, consider referring to child psychologist when binge eating or psychological problems are a big issue. Service provision varies between authorities. (See later in chapter for discussion of binge eating.)
- Offer regular follow–up with clear guidelines on discharge if goals are not being met.

Calcium

About 45% of adult skeletal mass is formed during adolescence (Bonjour, Theintz, Buchs, Slosman & Rizzoli 1991). Low bone density is related to the increased risk of osteoporosis in later life, especially in women (see Chapter 4, Health promotion). It is important to maximise calcium intake in adolescence as once the bone density peaks in the early 20s, little can be done to augment the calcium stored in the bone.

The recommended daily intake of calcium intake is as follows:

| Boys 11–18 | 1000 mg calcium |
| Girls 11–18 | 800 mg calcium |

Milk and milk products have a much higher concentration of calcium than other foods and the calcium from dairy foods is more readily absorbed than from other sources.

Approximately 60% of 14-year-old girls have an intake less than the recommended amount of calcium (Office of National Statistics 2000), therefore girls must be strongly encouraged to eat more calcium to protect their bones. Non-milk drinking young people need to be advised to consume other sources of calcium, for example soya milk and yoghurt, rice milk, white bread, cheese and tofu. Load-bearing exercise, such as walking, aids bone formation and is yet another good reason for promoting regular activity.

Iron

The recommended daily amount of iron is as follows:

| Boys 11–18 | 11.3 mg iron |
| Girls 11–18 | 14.8 mg iron |

This is achieved by eating food from meat, fish and alternatives group, bread and cereals group and vegetables.

Iron absorption is increased by the presence of haem iron, found in meats, and by vitamin C, found in citrus fruits. It is decreased by the presence of tea, coffee and the phytates in fibre. The most highly absorbed sources of iron are red meat and liver. Approximately 10% of 12–14 year old girls are anaemic, associated with a low dietary of iron and vitamin C (Nelson, Naismith, Burley, Gatenby & Geddesui 1990). As yet it is unclear whether anaemia causes poorer physical health, behaviour and academic performance. There is strong evidence that anaemia during pregnancy results in hypertension and heart disease in adulthood (Godfrey et al. 1991). It is worth considering the possibility of coeliac condition in young people whose anaemia doesn't obviously seem to be caused by low dietary iron intake.

Teenage pregnancy

Teenage pregnancy increases nutritional demands, especially if the mother herself is still growing. The major nutrients at risk are calcium, iron, zinc and folic acid. The four food groups provide all these. Food safety also requires careful consideration during pregnancy. Midwives have a special role to play developing the trust of teenage mothers and encouraging them to eat regularly and attend appointments. Many areas have groups for teenage mothers organised by specialist midwives and children's centres.

Vegetarianism

Vegetarianism has occurred throughout history for a variety of economic, religious, cultural and social reasons. Many parents are concerned when their child goes through a vegetarian phase, as they are unsure how to offer a balanced diet. A well-planned vegetarian eating pattern is a healthy way of eating as long as suitable alternatives to meat and fish are included. Unfortunately, some people who decide to stop eating meat also dislike vegetables, which is a challenge for the healthy balanced diet. Table 7.2 illustrates the nutrients that may be lacking in a vegetarian eating plan.

See Box 7.1 for suggestions for vegetarian sandwich fillings – try using different breads and wraps to increase variety and interest.

Table 7.2   The vegetarian way of eating – nutrients potentially at risk

Type of vegetarian	Nutrients that maybe at risk
No meat	Iron and zinc
No meat and fish	Iron, zinc. Omega-3 Polyunsaturated fats in oily fish
Vegans: no meat, fish, eggs or cows milk	Iron, zinc, omega-3 polyunsaturated fats in oily fish, vitaminB12, calcium, riboflavin
Macrobiotic/fruitarian diet	All of the above, protein, energy and trace elements

---

Box 7.1   Suggestions for sandwich fillings

- Grated cheese; mayonnaise and celery; cheese spreads with chutney or cranberry sauce; brie and grape; brie, basil and tomato; cheese and beetroot
- Cream cheese and cucumber; cream cheese; baby spinach and pine nuts
- Egg mayonnaise and sweetcorn
- Hummus and grated carrot; vegetable pate or bean spread with salad
- Peanut butter and banana; grated carrot; marmite and peanut butter
- Quorn slices with salad; vegetarian bacon slices with lettuce and tomato
- Red beans and salsa.

Meal ideas for a vegetarian in a non-vegetarian family

- Add beans (butter beans, chilli beans, lentils, black-eyed beans) to a portion of sauce for bolognaise, curry, chilli con carne or casserole before adding the meat
- Have rice dishes such as vegetable risotto with grated cheese, bean paella or vegetable pilau with lentils
- Use tinned beans such as red kidney beans, chick peas in pasta sauce or filling for jacket potato
- Vegetable stir fry with Quorn, tofu strips or nuts served with noodles or rice

- Eggs and cheese make quick meals such as omelette, cauliflower cheese, pasta and cheese sauce, cheese and potato pie, jacket potato with cheese and chives, cheese flans all served with vegetables
- Veggie burgers, vegetarian sausages and nut cutlets are handy alternatives to meat.

Sources of iron for vegetarians are from the egg, beans, lentils, dhal, nuts and seeds group of foods as well as bread and cereals, in particular fortified breakfast cereals and dark green vegetables. Sources of calcium for vegan and macrobiotic/fruitarian diets are soya milks, rice milks and oatmeal milks, which are fortified with calcium. This illustrates that choosing a mixture of foods from the four food groups at every meal ensures adequate nutrition.

The author has found that some Asian young people just eat vegetable dishes with chapatti, resulting in a low iron intake. Dhals (lentils) and beans such as chick peas are good sources of iron and protein and can be added to the vegetables.

Vitamin B12 is found only in animal foods, including eggs and milk. It is essential that young people choosing to eat vegan or macrobiotic diets include foods fortified with B12, such as most breakfast cereals, in their diet. Frank B12 deficiency causes megaloblastic anaemia; this is more commonly found among Asian vegetarians.

Activity 7.1

How would you advise a mother who is worried about her 14-year-old daughter who has recently given up eating meat, fish and eggs? Check your information leaflets – do you have support literature for this mother?

Food, health and low income

There are considerable differences in what people eat according to their income. People living in households without an earner consume more calories, fat, salt and sugar than those living in households with one or more earners (Office of National Statistics 2000). People on low incomes eat less variety of foods, mainly due to fear of potential waste (Dowler & Calvert 1995). They eat less fruit and vegetables, less milk, less fish and more processed foods. It is important to consider these issues when talking to young people and their families about their nutrition. It is also worth stressing that fresh fruit is often cheaper than junk food, for example, an apple is usually cheaper than a bar of chocolate or a packet of crisps.

School meals and national healthy school standard

School meals have undergone a major improvement in recent years, and more meals are now home cooked. The government increased funding from 2005, for three years, to raise the quality of school meals. This also includes the whole school approach to food by replacing fizzy pop with bottled water, and chocolate with healthy snacks, and by removing vending machines altogether. This is also applicable to tuck-shops. Nutrient based standards have been brought back by the government and come into force in 2008 for primary schools and 2009 for secondary schools (www.schoolfoodtrust.org. uk). The school food trust has been set up to provide independent support and advice. Your local council web site will have current information about the provision of local school meals.

The national healthy school standard (www.healthyschools.gov.uk) also influences promotion of healthy lifestyles within the school setting. It encompasses five objectives to promote healthy living including lifestyle, healthy eating, physical activity and emotional health and well-being within the school. The Department for Education and Skills (DfES) target is that every school achieves the standards by 2009.

Sports

The body's endogenous carbohydrate stores are used up after 60–90 minutes of moderate exercise. Therefore, young people who participate in high levels of sporting activity, such as dancing, football, boxing and swimming, need to pay attention to the following recommendations in order to maximise their performance:

- adequate carbohydrate intake: 60–70% of total energy intake. This can only be achieved by meals and frequent snacks every 1–2 hours;
- adequate fluid intake: aided by always carrying a sports bottle (full)
- timing to avoid long gaps between eating and exercise: eat high carbohydrate snacks after strenuous exercise. These include bread, cereal bars, breakfast cereals, bananas.

The biggest barrier to following these guidelines is a perceived lack of time, as these young people are usually very active.

Practice nurses have a challenge to help young people and their families address unhealthy eating patterns in order to attain optimum body weight for health and self-esteem.

Eating disorders

Eating disorders are not just about food or weight, but also about feelings. Sufferers are deeply distressed, with anorexia nervosa having one of the highest death rates of any mental disorder (Morgan & Treasure 2006). By concentrating all their energies on food and dieting, the eating disorder becomes a way of coping with emotional pain and turmoil. At first, dieting and weight loss provide a sense of achievement and control over one's life that gives relief from difficult feelings or intolerable dilemmas, but when the ill effects of starvation, frequent bingeing and/or purging become apparent, the eating disorder itself becomes the dominant problem and the sufferer feels trapped. This section explores the wider issues surrounding eating disorders, a condition that affects mainly younger women.

Definitions of eating disorders (American Psychiatric Association 1994)

Anorexia nervosa

The person refuses to maintain a body weight over a minimum normal weight for age and height, that is a body mass index ≤ 17.5, weighs less than 85% of predicted weight, or fails to make an expected weight gain during a period of growth. They have an intense fear of gaining weight or becoming fat even though underweight, and over-evaluate their shape and weight, or deny the seriousness of low body weight. Females may have an absence of at least three consecutive menstrual cycles when otherwise expected to occur (primary or secondary amenorrhoea), unless taking a contraceptive, while men may have reduced libido.

Bulimia nervosa

Bulimia nervosa is suggested by recurrent episodes of binge eating, an episode of binge eating being characterised by eating in a discrete period of time (e.g. any 2-hour period) an amount of food that is definitely larger than most people would eat during a similar period of time in similar circumstances, the most common foods on which to binge being sweet high-calorie foods such as ice cream, cakes, chocolate and biscuits.

The sufferer will also have:

1. a sense of lack of control over eating during the episode, for example, a feeling that one cannot stop or control how much one is eating
2. recurrent compensatory behaviour in order to prevent weight gain, for example, self-induced vomiting, laxative abuse, the use of other drugs such as diuretics, fasting or excessive exercise
3. a minimum average of two binge eating and inappropriate compensatory behaviours per week for at least three months
4. a tendency to leave the table immediately after a meal and disappearing to the toilet in order to vomit food eaten.

Binge eating disorder

All the criteria for bulimia nervosa are met except that the compensatory behaviour (see '2' above) is absent or infrequent. This usually leads to significant weight gain (Young & Root 2006).

It is possible to have a mixture of the features described above and the sufferer may, in the course of time, move from one eating disorder to another. It is also possible to have some, but not all, of the features; these are called partial syndromes or defined as EDNOS (Eating Disorders Not Otherwise Specified). It is thought that they may be more common than the full disorders. Binge eating disorder (BED) may not always be recognised as a true eating disorder.

Activity 7.2

Check when the practice weighing scales were last serviced. If not included in an annual service contract, discuss this with the practice team at your next meeting.

Prevalence

There have been numerous studies that have estimated the prevalence rates of anorexia nervosa (AN) and bulimia nervosa (BN). Wide variations have been reported due to the relative rarity of eating disorders, the reluctance of sufferers to participate in surveys and the fluctuating nature of the illness; the latter posing difficulties in interpretation of symptoms.

However, according to (Morgan & Treasure 2006) the average GP list that includes 2000 patients at any one time is likely to have:

- 1–2 patients with AN
- 18 patients with BN

Approximately 5–10% of teenage girls will have some degree of disordered eating, and may be using weight-reducing techniques other than dieting, such as vomiting, laxative or diuretic abuse or excessive exercising.

Increasing numbers of people with eating disorders are being identified. Young and Root (2006) report the greatest increase in incidence rates is among young females aged 10–19 years. Onset for AN is around 15–24 years and peaks at 18 years, but can occur at any age, with children as young as nine reported to be dieting (Raisingkids 2005). A prevalence of 0.7% in teenage girls has been given (Fairburn & Harrison 2003). A third of anorexics are reported to be overweight as children, with a rise in the number of boys being diagnosed (Raisingkids 2005). It has been suggested that 10–20% of all cases may be male (Young & Root 2006).

BN often goes undiagnosed and untreated, but an incidence of 0.5–1% of young women has been given by NHS Direct (2006), while Hay (2007) gives a figure of 1–2% sufferers in young Western women. Over 85% of reported cases of BN occur in girls in their late teens and early 20s (NHS Direct 2006).

Men

Approximately 10% of men suffer from BN (NHS Direct 2006) and AN (Morgan & Treasure 2006). An increasing number of men are coming forward for treatment, although men are more likely to be under diagnosed, misdiagnosed and under-referred, and less likely to be referred to top specialist services for treatment than women (Morgan & Treasure 2006).

Although there are no available figures for BED, atypical eating disorders, which include BED, may affect more than half of people with an eating disorder (National Institute for Clinical Excellence 2004).

Presenting symptoms at the surgery

Although the individual may present for a wide variety of medical conditions, common symptoms relate to the effects of starvation and purging behaviour. The young person with an eating disorder may present with a range of symptoms (Boxes 7.2 and 7.3). The keen observational skills of the nurse, in addition to a good rapport with the patient during a consultation for any reason, are an opportunity to recognise a potential eating disorder.

Box 7.2   Signs and symptoms of anorexia nervosa (Morgan & Treasure 2006; Raisingkids 2005)

- Fear of normal body weight
- Lack of concern about low weight
- Distortion of body image
- Judging themselves solely in terms of weight and shape
- Over exercise
- Severely restricted food intake
- Fatigue
- Altered sleep cycle
- Sensitivity to cold; may have signs and symptoms of Raynaud's disease
- Dizziness
- Psychosocial problems
- Dental caries
- Sore throat
- Abdominal symptoms – constipation, fullness after eating
- Sub fertility, amenorrhoea (if they are not taking an oral contraceptive)
- Dry skin, brittle nails
- Growth of downy hair may appear on face

Box 7.3   Signs and symptoms of bulimia nervosa (NHS Direct 2006, Hay 2007)

- Fluctuations in weight
- Sore throat, heartburn and dental caries caused by excessive vomiting
- Puffiness of the face caused by swollen salivary glands
- Acne and poor skin condition
- Scarred knuckles due to attempts to force fingers down the throat to induce vomiting
- Irregulars menses
- Lethargy and tiredness
- Depression, anxiety, low self-esteem and mood swings
- Constipation and intestinal damage
- Regular binge eating
- Preoccupation with food and diet

Anorexia nervosa

The anorexic is unlikely to come forward and ask for help. As sufferers see it, there is nothing wrong (the eating disorder has cured the problem), and so no treatment is necessary. They usually see themselves as being too fat and will be trying to lose more weight. Sufferers are often brought to the attention of medical services by relatives alarmed at food refusal and weight loss.

When the disorder is well established the general appearance is one of emaciation. Low weight in recent onset AN may be less obvious and change in weight or rate of weight loss may be more pertinent. Other symptoms to look out for are related to biological adaptations to starvation, including amenorrhoea, feeling the cold, low blood pressure, tiredness and weakness.

There are many illnesses in which poor appetite and consequently poor food intake may cause severe weight loss. It is important to establish whether there is a deliberate attempt to restrict food intake in order to lose weight before AN can be suspected.

Bulimia nervosa

BN has been described as a secret disorder and unless the sufferer discloses their problem, it can lie undetected for many years. Outwardly the person is usually within the normal weight range and trying to follow a healthy lifestyle. They may present at the general practice surgery with symptoms related to the purging behaviour; for example; abdominal pain, mouth ulcers and oesophagitis. Occasionally the complaint is of an inability to diet due to compulsive eating (bingeing). Severe vomiting and laxative abuse can lead to major fluid and electrolyte disturbances which may need emergency treatment. Depression is more common in BN than AN.

Binge eating disorder

Sufferers are usually overweight and binge on large quantities of food in response to emotional stress; for example, exams, loneliness, bullying. This bingeing is a much more compulsive activity than eating for comfort or boredom and has to be distinguished from these. Young people with binge eating disorders are much more likely to be referred to a dietician or the practice nurse for weight management than be diagnosed as a sufferer of an eating disorder.

Causes

There is no single cause but the commonly found contributory factors are summarised in Box 7.4.

Box 7.4   Contributory factors in eating disorders (Hay 2007; NHS Direct 2006)

Life events:

- Death of a close relative or friend
- Illness of a parent - mental or physical
- Divorce or separation of parents
- Leaving home
- Termination of pregnancy
- Sexual or physical abuse, or neglect
- Ending of a close relationship
- Examinations
- Bullying or teasing
- Onset of menstruation.

Cultural/social influences:

- Fashion industry
- Social pressures to be thin and the stigma of being fat
- Critical comments about weight or body shape, or both.

Low self-esteem:

- Many sufferers feel a lack of self worth, sometimes to the point of self loathing.

Personality:

- Perfectionist
- Obsessional, e.g. with tidiness, cleanliness and appearance
- High, often unrealistic, expectations of achievements
- Compliant and quiet child, prior to onset of eating disorder.

Family:

- Difficulty in dealing with problems
- Excessive concern about body shape, weight or fitness, and dieting
- Alcohol misuse
- Parental and childhood obesity
- Parental and pre-morbid psychiatric disorder
- Parental problems, such as high expectations, low care and overprotection
- A possible genetic link.

Treatment and outcome

Most sufferers can be treated on an outpatient basis. Only very severe cases will need admission to hospital. The mainstays of treatment for eating disorders are:

- education about eating disorders
- counselling and psychotherapy (cognitive behaviour therapy)
- family therapy
- nutritional counselling.

Specialised services and units may also provide a range of other treatments such as life skills, creative therapies and relaxation programmes. The sooner treatment starts after the onset of the eating disorder, the better the outcome. The practice nurse is well placed to help sufferers and their families, but there is good evidence that treatment must be at the right time as well as appropriate. It is likely that the sufferer will eventually need to be referred to a therapist or specialist service with experience in dealing with eating disorders. However, there is much that the practice nurse can do to help.

Practice nurse involvement

As specialist service provision is limited, practice nurses can identify and manage some patients, using their expertise in dietary advice, basic counselling skills and arranging monitoring of the physical aspects of patient care (Young & Root 2006). The patient may present with a range of complaints (see Boxes 7.2 and 7.3) before disclosing their eating disorder.

Engage the patient in treatment

The first step is to help sufferers to *acknowledge* they have a problem and that it is psychological in origin. This may take a few sessions but it is time well spent. Many sufferers will deny they have a problem or play down the seriousness of it and so will not be receptive to treatment if it is offered too soon.

The next step is to *educate* the patient (and the family) about eating disorders. See the useful addresses section for helpful literature. Encourage them to join the Eating Disorders Association and/or a self-help group (if your area has one). Some people get better without further help once given relevant information.

Teaching sufferers about the ill effects of starving and purging and their medical consequences, in both the short and long term, is also helpful, as

Table 7.3 Serious complications of eating disorders (Morgan & Treasure 2006; NHS Direct 2006)

Eating disorder	Complication	Cause
Bulimia	Dental erosion	Contact with stomach acid
	Swollen, torn or irritated oesophagus	From vomiting
	Cardiac problems, occasionally death	Electrolyte imbalance and dehydration
	Rupture of stomach	Bingeing
Anorexia nervosa	Severe dehydration or overhydration, acute renal failure, electrolyte imbalance	Vomiting and diuretic and laxative abuse
	Osteoporosis	Prolonged poor nutrition during critical development of peak bone mass

many people do not realise the damage caused by their eating disorder (see Table 7.3).

The third step is to *motivate* the patient to want to recover and make changes. Treatment involves facing up to the difficulties that the eating disorder has resolved, so it can be a long, painful and sometimes frightening experience. Explaining that treatment will involve talking about feelings as well as the eating problems is helpful in preparing them for therapy.

Finally, *reassure* the patient, but pay special attention to their family; the anxiety generated by them often makes matters worse. Try to help them to concentrate on talking to their family and friends about their problems, rather than battling over food.

Activity 7.3

Find out the details of the nearest self-help group for Eating Disorders, and post it on the practice website and/or the surgery notice board in a visible position.

Practical measures

A full medical examination is essential to assess current health status and exclude other causes of weight loss/gain, and needs to include:

- a history of the patient's eating habits
- calculation of body mass index (BMI) plotted on a percentile chart, noting weight changes

---

Box 7.5   SCOFF questionnaire

A 'Yes' to two or more questions suggests the patient has an eating disorder

1. Do you ever make yourself **S**ick because you feel uncomfortably full?
2. Do you worry you have lost **C**ontrol over how much you eat?
3. Have you recently lost more than **O**ne stone in a three month period?
4. Do you believe yourself to be **F**at when others say you are too thin?
5. Would you say that **F**ood dominates your life?

- biochemistry (urea and electrolytes and blood glucose, thyroid function)
- haematology (white cell count and haemoglobin level)
- physical examination including blood pressure
- other signs of self-harm, for example: alcohol or drug misuse, cutting, suicide attempts, suicidal thoughts
- use of the SCOFF questionnaire as a screening tool (see Box 7.5).

The following findings need to be referred to the general practitioner and acted on quickly:

- a very low weight (a BMI <15)
- any serious drop in weight (1kg per week over 8 weeks)
- escalating purging behaviour
- suicidal intentions.

Referral

A practice counsellor, with or without the support of a dietician, may be able to help in many mild cases. A specific cognitive behavioural psychotherapy has been developed for BN, which has been found to be acceptable to sufferers, reducing symptoms of BN and depression (Hay 2007). Interpersonal therapy may be offered if CBT is unsuccessful (National Institute for Clinical Excellence 2004). The range of options for AN includes cognitive analytic therapy, cognitive behaviour therapy, interpersonal therapy, and family therapy (National Institute for Clinical Excellence 2004). More severe and/or complicated cases may need referral for specialist advice.

Referrals out of the practice will depend on availability of local services, specialist teams and eating disorders units (either NHS or private). A third of health authorities have no local specialist provision (Young & Root 2006). Child and adolescent services will accept young people who are still at school. The Eating Disorders Association has a database of specialist services (see resources.)

Activity 7.4

Liaise with your primary healthcare team colleagues to find out what local mental health services are available for eating disorders, and how to refer sufferers. Add to your contact address book.

Very low weight individuals (with a BMI less than15), and those with severe electrolyte disturbances, will need urgent medical attention, and hospital admission may need to be considered. Practice nurses may be the first point of contact for sufferers of eating disorders, and must be alert to the potential sufferer when asked to advise on weight and diet, or through their observational skills. Some patients can be successfully managed in general practice, but a knowledge of local services and methods of referral is essential for ensuring that these patients receive the specialist help they deserve.

Teenage healthcare

Many young people have no interest in their health, which makes the health professional's role extremely challenging. To them, ill health occurs in old age; that is, in their parents and those over 40! Promoting healthy lifestyles for young people will reduce morbidity and premature mortality, although the effects of health education cannot always be assessed in the short term.

One teenage male patient said 'Well, I don't want to get old anyway, so I'll enjoy myself now'. As parents, many readers will relate to this comment and appreciate the difficulties of approaching teenage health issues.

Health promotion will often be opportunistic when the young person presents with an acute problem or for routine immunisations or travel advice, and will supplement advice already given in school or at home. Others will attend specifically for advice. Parents appear less enthusiastic to discuss sexual health with their children, perhaps because they hope that the need will not arise. Practice nurses can fill this void through informed and sensitive advice and support. The following text emphasises the rationale for young peoples' health needs to be included in any health agenda but leaves it to the reader to plan the approach best suited to each locality. The main emphasis is on sexual health, but issues relating to confidentiality and access relate to all areas of health.

Every child matters

Every Child Matters (DfES 2003) and the Children's Act 2004 aim to safeguard and promote the welfare of children through multiagency working. This includes all aspects of health and recognises young people's sexuality. *Healthy Schools* (DfES 2003) aims to improve health and reduce inequalities, raise pupil achievement, have more social inclusion and have closer working between health promotion providers and schools. Sex and relationship education must include information on the links between recreational drugs, alcohol and unsafe sex. It should be delivered in schools as part of personal, social and health education (PHSE) sessions and linked to lifestyle issues.

Recreational drugs and alcohol

Alcohol consumption in young people rose to 11.3 units (boys) and 10.3 units (girls) per week in 2004, almost double that consumed in 1990 (National Centre for Social Research/National Foundation for Education Research 2005). Alcohol consumption has been cited as the main reason for first intercourse in 13% of young women and 20% of young men aged 15–19 (Wellings et al. 1994 cited by brook 2007). Alcohol consumption becomes more common with age in young people. It is reported that 23% of 11–15 year olds drank, rising to 45% of 15 year olds (NCSR 2005). Recreational drug usage also rises with age and its use has been associated with unsafe sex. The National Centre for Social Research/National Foundation for Education Research (2005) stated that 1% of 11 year olds use cannabis, rising to 26% of 15 year olds. These figures are pertinent when considered with first age of intercourse (see later).

Many areas of health promotion are included within the National Curriculum and are discussed in PHSE throughout a child's education. Practice nurses who offer a sensitive, confidential health clinic, can fill gaps in this provision.

Young person's clinic

Healthcare can be delivered either opportunistically, in a planned appointment, or in a clinic environment. Specific clinics for teenagers are difficult to establish, but some young people do respond to the interest of health workers, particularly if they have a specific problem that needs addressing Local needs must be identified before attempting to establish a young person's clinic within general practice; provision and energies can then be directed appropriately (see Chapter 4). Clinics can be run either by invitation or as a drop-in service. A drop-in facility enables any emergency (for example, emergency contraceptive needs) to be dealt with immediately. Some young people want to access services within school hours, particularly if they are dependent on school transport. Others will prefer after school services. Flexibility is essential to deliver needs-driven service.

The many issues that the nurse and/or young person may wish to discuss are listed in Box 7.6. General lifestyle advice relating to smoking, alcohol, diet and exercise is pertinent to everyone, regardless of age, and should be tailored to the individual. It would also be naive to exclude recreational drugs and sexual health from the agenda. Any young person who uses recreational drugs or consumes alcohol may require specialist help and referral to a drug and alcohol agency.

Health professionals must be alert to girls who exercise excessively and/or have low dietary calcium, both of which are recognised risk factors for development of osteoporosis. Eating disorders were discussed earlier in the chapter.

Box 7.6   Health issues for young people

The many health issues pertinent to young people include:

- current health status
- smoking status
- alcohol consumption
- recreational drugs
- exercise: amount and type
- dietary advice: weight control, vegetarian, calcium intake
- family history: hyperlipidaemia, coronary heart disease, breast or cervical cancer, testicular cancer
- breast awareness (girls)
- testicular self-examination (boys)
- acne
- relationship problems
- bullying
- school pressures
- sexual health: contraception and emergency contraception, sexually transmitted diseases, safer sex and sexuality
- any 'taboo' topics the person may not wish to discuss with family or peers

---

It is essential that the nurse can make the young person feel comfortable to gain their confidence. Mental health issues require more specialist advice. These should be referred to the psychiatric services.

Confidentiality

The young person has to be sure that the nurse will maintain confidentiality (see Chapter 1). One of the main deterrents regarding seeking help and advice is a fear of lack of confidentiality and fear of being told off (Brook 2007a). This appears to outweigh their fear of pregnancy or sexually transmitted diseases.

The duty of confidentiality to any person under the age of 16 is as great as that for any adult. Children aged under 16 who are able to fully understand proposed treatment and its implications are competent to consent to medical treatment regardless of age. The nurse is, however, legally obliged to discuss the value of parental involvement and encourage the young person to inform a parent. If the child declines they must be assured that their confidentiality will be respected.

Young people who are made aware of these issues may be more confident to approach health professionals for health or contraceptive advice. This is perhaps the fundamental hurdle that must be overcome before a substantial reduction in teenage pregnancy will be seen.

Teenage sexual health clinic

General practices should offer a nonjudgemental sexual health service for those young people who require advice and support. The many consequences of early sexual activity are listed in Box 7.7.

Box 7.7   Consequences of early sexual activity

These include:

- sexually transmitted diseases, including HIV, hepatitis B, genital herpes
- unplanned pregnancy (see Chapter 4, preconceptual care)
- cervical neoplasia
- exploitation
- psychological trauma

Sex education is a vital element in the care of both the sexually active and the teenager contemplating sexual activity. A teenage sexual health clinic should have clear aims, which may include:

- providing a user-friendly environment
- providing user-friendly terminology
- giving holistic advice regarding aspects of general healthcare
- encouraging responsibility in sexual matters
- stressing that confidentiality is maintained.

Sexual health is an important issue at any age but the teenage years are of special importance to ensure a healthy and well-informed adult population. This was included as a *Health of the Nation* target, which aimed to reduce the rate of conceptions among under 16s by at least 50% by the year 2000 – from 9.5 per 1000 girls aged 13–15 years in 1989 to no more than 4.8 per 1000 girls (Department of Health 1992). Although this target was excluded from *Our Healthier Nation* (Department of Health 1998), health workers must continue their efforts to reduce schoolgirl conceptions.

Fraser guidelines give specific guidance regarding the provision of advice and treatment for young people under the age of 16 years (Brook 2007b). If these guidelines are followed sexual health services can be delivered without parental consent. If the nurse is concerned that a young person is being abused a referral must be made via the local Child Protection services.

It has been shown that since 1990 first intercourse is now taking place at a younger age, a greater proportion of people have multiple partners and a greater proportion of men have had a same-sex partner (Johnson et al. 2001). This has implications for both conceptions and the risk of contracting STIs.

Sexually transmitted infections

The new National Institute for Clinical Excellence guidelines (2007) recommend one-to-one interventions to reduce the transmission of sexually transmitted infections (STIs) and under 18 conceptions, especially in the vulnerable and at-risk groups. Sexual health has deteriorated in the past 12 years, resulting in large increases in many STIs. Females aged 16–19 and males aged 20–24 have the highest rates of chlamydia, with numbers increasing by 3% and 7% respectively since the mid 1990s (Health Protection Agency 2006a). The number of cases of gonorrhoea diagnosed in GUM clinics in the UK has increased by 111% between 1195 and 2004, with the same age distribution as chlamydia (Health Protection Agency 2006b). Nurses can advertise, either by posters or word of mouth, that free condoms are available in the practice or local family planning clinic in an attempt to promote safer sex, and refer patients to the genito-urinary clinic if full STI screening is required.

Teenage pregnancy

Under 18 and under 16 conception rates in England have fallen by 11.1% and 15.2% respectively since the inception of the Teenage Pregnancy strategy in 1998, and are now at their lowest level for 20 years (Teenage Pregnancy Unit 2006). Despite this reduction, teenage pregnancy rates in the UK remain the highest in the Western world. These statistics are encouraging but highlight the ever present need to educate and support young people in all aspects of sexual health.

Risk factors associated with teenage pregnancy

Teenage pregnancy is 10 times more likely to occur in girls whose parents are in social group V than those whose parents are professional (Brook 2007c). Other risk factors for teenage pregnancy are listed in Box 7.8.

Approximately 25% of girls who have been in care are mothers by the age of 16 and almost 50% are mothers 18–24 months after leaving care (Brook 2007c).

Box 7.8   Risk factors for teenage pregnancy (Department for Education and Skills 2006)

Factors that increase the likelihood of teenage pregnancy include:

Risky behaviours

- Early onset of sexual activity
- Poor contraceptive use
- Mental health disorders and conduct disorders and or involvement in crime
- Alcohol and substance misuse
- Already a teenage mother or had a termination

Educational factors

- Low educational attainment or no qualifications
- Disengagement from school

Family background

- Living in care
- Daughter of a teenage mother
- Daughter of a mother who has low educational aspirations for them
- Belonging to a particular ethnic group

The three major factors identified in the *Report on Teenage Pregnancy* (Social Exclusion Unit 1999) in its search for the UK's failure to reduce teenage conceptions compared with other European countries are:

1. Low expectations – disadvantaged young people who have low educational or employment expectations
2. Ignorance – a lack of accurate knowledge of sexually transmitted infections and contraception
3. Mixed messages – sexual images and sexual messages surround young people implying the sexual activity is the normal, but young people note that parents or public institutions find dealing with young people's sexuality uncomfortable so it is often not dealt with adequately.

Daughters of mothers who had a teenage pregnancy appear more likely to become teenage mothers themselves (Seamark & Gray 1997). A small controlled study supporting this theory involved 31 girls who had had at least one teenage pregnancy. The mother's pregnancy history was also established. The planned pregnancies were not terminated (Table 7.4).

Outcomes associated with teenage pregnancy

Over 50% of pregnant 13–15 year olds and 40% of 15–19 year olds will have their pregnancy terminated, while those who continue their pregnancy and become teenage parents tend to have poor ante-natal health, lower birth weight babies and higher infant mortality rates, and their children's health is often poorer than average (Brook 2007c). Becoming a parent is a positive outcome for some young people, but more often teenage pregnancy is associated with poor social outcomes and poor health for both mother and child. Young mothers are less likely to breastfeed, more likely to suffer postnatal depression, often do not finish their education and live in poverty (Botting, Rosato & Wood 1998).

The health of the young teenage mother is compromised by obstetric complications, including hypertension, anaemia, placental abruption and

Table 7.4 A study into teenage pregnancy (Seamark & Gray 1997)

Mother had teenage pregnancy				
	pregnancy number	planned	continued	terminated
yes	16	5	5	6
no	15	1	2	12

depression. Termination of pregnancy has its own associated physical and psychological problems. Social inclusion aims to reduce the gaps in a teenage girl's education, thus improving long term-employment prospects (Department for Education and Skills 2003).

Activity 7.5

Discuss the numbers of under-16 pregnancies within your practice with your attached midwife. Has the number increased or decreased over the past two years? Is it possible to identify pregnancies related to method failure and those due to inaccessibility of sexual health services? Consider the implications of your findings.

Prevention of teenage pregnancy

Attitudes towards teenage sexuality must be open and accepting and there should be appropriate sex and relationship education, easy access to confidential contraceptive services and information widely available. Within general practice, facilities exist for young people to access confidential help and advice regarding all aspects of sexual health, contraception and emergency contraception, the most accessible and appropriate person being the family planning trained practice nurse.

Research has highlighted that regardless of from whom or from where young people get their sex education, a very important aspect to consider is *when* it is given. It has been demonstrated that changing sexual and contraceptive behaviour is less successful when young people have already commenced sexual activity before the programme starts (NHS Centre for Reviews and Dissemination 1997).

It is vital that young people are aware of the availability of emergency contraception and know when and from where they can obtain it. Emergency contraception has been available without prescription, but at a cost, from pharmacies since January 2001, although some pharmacies do dispense it under a Patient Group Direction (see Chapter 9) (Brook 2007d).

Emergency contraception is an extremely effective and safe method of avoiding pregnancy following unprotected intercourse or method failure. This can be either hormonal (emergency contraceptive pills) or the intra-uterine device (IUD). The former is the most common method used for the young person as insertion of an IUD may prove difficult in a young woman who has not been pregnant, and is unsuitable for those at high risk of sexually transmitted disease. However, the risk of unintended pregnancy should

---

Box 7.9   Barriers to young people accessing services (Graham, Green & Glasier 1996)

The young person:

- may not know where to find family planning services
- may not have the confidence to insist on an emergency appointment
- may be unaware of confidentiality.

Clinic times may not be outside school hours therefore access will be difficult.

---

be weighed against these risks, notably because the IUD is so effective. Even when the young woman has knowledge of emergency contraception, she may find it difficult to obtain it for several reasons (Box 7.9).

General practices can provide contraceptive services to girls who are registered elsewhere. This knowledge may increase uptake of contraceptive services, as confidentiality is often a girl's major concern.

Activity 7.6

Discuss with colleagues and service users how contraceptive services within your practice could be more 'user friendly' to encourage young people to access the services.

Boys, young men

It would appear from the above text that sexual health advice and contraception are the domain of girls, but young men also have a responsibility to prevent pregnancy and to reduce the spread of STIs. This should be considered in all health promotion initiatives.

Men are poor users of health services, as noted in Chapter 5, and are often reluctant to ask for or accept help (Lloyd & Forest 2001). They view sexual health services as being for girls/women (Brook 2007e). Previous research showed that boys in particular have low levels of knowledge about contraception, reproduction and contraceptive services (Winn, Roker & Coleman 1995). They still appear to be less likely than girls to know where or how to access services (Balding 2005). Boys are said to consider that issues of contraception and pregnancy are the responsibility of girls, and feel it is irrelevant to them (Brook 2007e). An early survey of 16–19-year-old young men reported the main source of sex information to be from school lessons (Wellings et al. 2001, cited by Brook 2007e). A later study by Balding (2005) stated that friends were the main source of sex information. Brook figures (2007d) noted an increase of 215% during 1996–2000 and 14% during 2005–2006 in young men aged under 25 years accessing their clinics. The increase in access to community clinics is still significant, at 43%.

As noted in Chapter 5, issues relating to sexuality also need addressing when a young man is confused about his own sexuality. This highlights the importance of sex education for both boys and girls to prevent sexually transmitted infections as well as pregnancies. Encouraging boys to attend family planning or sexual health clinics would offer an opportunity to discuss all aspects of sexuality, sexually transmitted diseases and contraception.

Young men often lead lifestyles that make their parents despair. They ignore advice on healthy eating, smoking, alcohol consumption, recreational drugs and general health. Health professionals must try to tailor their advice to suit the lifestyles of modern youth, in an effort to promote physical, mental and sexual health.

Summary

Young people are bombarded with conflicting messages from the media, advertisements, family and health professionals. The importance of good nutrition in childhood cannot be overstated. Obese children will often remain overweight in adulthood, with all the associated health risks. The nurse can advise, guide and support young people to follow a healthy eating pattern that may be alien to the family, but still include all the necessary nutrients for growth and health. This must be undertaken in such a way that it does not lead to the young person developing an eating disorder. Most people with eating disorders will recover, but a small proportion of people become chronic sufferers or die from the effects of starvation or suicide. Specialist referral is essential for these people.

Young people have similar health needs to adults but access to, and delivery of, these services needs special consideration. Raising the subject of a confidential service for young people during routine immunisations can be a useful introduction to a young people's clinic. The young person must be treated with respect, reassured about confidentiality and offered sound, accurate information. The nurse has a responsibility to liaise with colleagues and other agencies if concerned about any aspect of a young person's safety.

The challenge is to motivate lifestyle changes, offer support and know when to refer to other agencies. This requires the skills of the practice nurse to enhance the young person's self-esteem in all aspects of their life.

Key points

- Healthy eating patterns start in childhood
- Obese children will often grow up to obese adults
- Young people have their own health needs
- Confidentiality must be respected
- The sexual health of young men must be included in a health agenda

Recommended reading

Basari ME. (2002) *Human Nutrition A Health Perspective.* London: Arnold.
Buttriss J, Wynne A & Stanner S (2001) *Nutrition. A Handbook for Community Nurses.* London: Whurr.
Includes recommendations for nutrition throughout life.
Mann J & Truswell S (2002) *Essentials of Human Nutrition.* Oxford: Oxford University Press.
National Institute for Health and Clinical Excellence (2004) *Eating Disorders: Core Interventions in the Treatment and Management of Anorexia Nervosa, Bulimia Nervosa and Related Eating Disorders.* London: NICE. www.nice.org.uk
Palmer RL (1996) *Understanding Eating Disorders.* London: Family Doctor Publications.
Treasure J (1997) *Anorexia Nervosa: A Survival Guide for Families, Friends and Sufferers.* London: Psychology Press.

References

American Psychiatric Association (1994) *Diagnostic and Statistical Manual of Mental Disorders 4th edn.* Washington DC: American Psychiatric Association.
Balding J (2005) *Young People in 2004.* www.sheu.org.uk
Botting B, Rosato M & Wood R (1998) Teenage mothers and the health of their children. ONS *Population Trends* 93, 19–28.
Bonjour JP, Theintz G, Buchs B, Slosman D & Rizzoli R (1991) Critical years and stages of puberty for spinal and femoral bone mass accumulation during adolescence. *Journal of Clinical Endocrinology and Metabolism* 73, 55.
Brook (2007a) *Brook's Position on Confidentiality.* www.brook.org.uk/content/M6_4_confidentiality.asp.

Brook (2007b) *Brook's Position on Under Sixteens.* www.brook.org.uk/content/M6_4_ undersixteens.asp.

Brook (2007c) *Brook's Position on Teenage Pregnancy.* www.brook.org.uk/content/M6_ 4_teenage%20pregnancy.asp.

Brook (2007d) *Brook's Position on Emergency Contraception.* www.brook.org.uk/ content/M6_4_emergencycontracpetion.asp.

Brook (2007e) *Brook's Position on Boys and Young Men.* www.brook.org.uk/content/ M6_4_boysandyoungmen.asp.

Department for Education and Skills (2003) *Every Child Matters.* www. everychildmatters.gov.uk.

Department for Education and Skills (2006) *Teenage Pregnancy: Accelerating the Strategy for 2010.* London: DfES.

Department of Health (1992) *The Health of the Nation: A Strategy for Health in England.* London: HMSO.

Department of Health (1998) *Our Healthier Nation. A Summary of the Consultation Paper.* London: HMSO.

Department of Health (2004) *At Least Five a Week: Evidence of the Impact of Physical Activity and it Relationship to Health. A Report from the Chief Medical Officer.* London: DH.

Dowler E & Calvert C (1995) *Nutrition and Diet in Lone Parent Families in London.* London: Family Policies Study Centre.

Fairburn CG & Harrison PJ (2003) Eating disorders. *Lancet* 361, 407–416.

Godfrey KM, Redman CWG, Barker DJP &Osmond C (1991) The effect of maternal anaemia and iron deficiency on the ratio of fetal weight to placental weight. *British Journal of Obstetrics and Gynaecology* 98, 886–891.

Graham A, Green L & Glasier F (1996) Teenagers knowledge of emergency contraception: questionnaire survey in South East Scotland. *British Medical Journal* 312, 1567–1569.

Hancox RJ, Milne BJ & Poulton R (2004) Association between child and adolescent television viewing and adult health: a longitudinal cohort study. *Lancet* 364, 257–262.

Hay P (2007) *Bulimia nervosa: diagnosis and treatment* (Just in time). www.bmjlearning. com/planrecord/servlet/ResourceSearchServlet?keyword=bu (accessed 8 January 2007).

Health Protection Agency (2006a) *Epidemiological data – Chlamydia.* www.hpa.org.uk.

Health Protection Agency (2006b) *Epidemiological data – Gonorrhoea.* www.hpa.org. uk.

Health Survey (2004) *Updating of the Trends Tables to Include Childhood Obesity Data.* www.ic.nhs.uk/pubs/hsechildobesityupdate.

Johnson AM, Mercer CD, Erens B et al. (2001) Sexual health in Britain: partnerships, practices and HIV risk behaviours. *Lancet* 358(9296), 1835–1842.

Lloyd T & Forest S (2001) *Boys and Young Men. Literature and Practice Review.* London: Health Development Agency.

Morgan J & Treasure J (2006) *Anorexia Nervosa: Diagnosis and Treatment* (Just in time). www.bmjlearning.com/planrecord/servlet/ResourceSearchServlet?keyword=an (accessed 14 October 2006).

National Centre for Social Research/National Foundation for Education Research (2005) *Drug Use, Smoking and Drinking Among Young People in England in 2004.* www.natcen.ac.uk.

NHS Centre for Reviews and Dissemination (1997) Preventing and reducing the adverse effects of unintended teenage pregnancies. *Effective Healthcare* 3(1), 1–12.

NHS Direct (2006) *Bulimia.* www.nhsdirect.nhs.uk/articles/article.aspx?articleId=68 (accessed 14 October 2006).

National Institute for Clinical Excellence (2004) *Eating Disorders: Anorexia Nervosa, Bulimia Nervosa and Related Eating Disorders. Understanding NICE guidance: a guide for people with eating disorders, their advocates and carers, and the public.* London: NICE.

National Institute for Clinical Excellence (2006) *NICE Guidelines on Obesity. CG43.* www.nice.org.uk.

National Institute for Clinical Excellence (2007) *One to One Intervention to Reduce the Transmission of Sexually Transmitted Infections (STIs) Including HIV, and to Reduce the Rate of Under-18 Conceptions, Especially those in Vulnerable and at Risk Groups.* www.nice.org.uk.

Nelson M, Naismith DJ, Burley V, Gatenby S & Geddes N (1990) Nutrient intakes, vitamin-mineral supplementation and intelligence in British schoolchildren. *British Journal of Nutrition* 64, 13–22.

Office of National Statistics (2000) *National Diet and Nutrition Survey 2000.* www.ons.gov.uk.

Raisingkids (2005) *Anorexia and your Teenager.* www.raisingkids.co.uk (accessed 20 May 2005).

Rudolph M, Christie D, Cellophane S, Shoat P, Dicey R, Walker J & Welling C (2006) Watch it: a community based programme for obese children and adolescents. *Archive of Diseases of Childhood* 91, 736–739.

Seamark C & Gray D (1997) Like mother, like daughter: a general practice study of maternal influences on teenage pregnancy *British Journal of General Practice* 47, 175–176.

Social Exclusion Unit (1999) *Social Exclusion Report on Teenage Pregnancies.* www.dfes.gov.uk.

Taheri S (2006) The link between short sleep duration and obesity: we should recommend more sleep to prevent obesity. *Archives of Diseases of Childhood* 91, 881–884.

Teenage Pregnancy Unit (2006) *Under-18 Conception Data for Top Tier Local Authorities LAD2. 1998–2004.* www.dfes.gov.uk.

Winn S, Roker D & Coleman J (1995) Knowledge about puberty and sexual development in 11–16 year old: implications for health and sex education in schools *Educational Studies* 21, 187–201.

Young M & Root H (2006) Identifying and treating eating disorders in primary care. *Independent Nurse* Feb 6. 14–15.

Useful addresses

British Dietetic Association
5th Floor, Charles House

148–9 Great Charles Street
Queensway
Birmingham B3 3HT.
www.bda.uk.com
Fact sheets and paediatric group diet information.

Brook
www.brook.org.uk
Provides free and confidential sexual health services and advice for young
people under 25.

Child Growth Foundation
2 Mayfield Avenue
London W4 1PW
Tel: 020 8995 0257 020 8994 7625
www.childgrowthfoundation.org.uk

BMI and waist circumference chart based on 1990 UK BMI reference curves.
Designed and published by Child growth Foundation. Supplied by Harlow
Printing Ltd.

DOH publications order lines
PO Box 777
London SE1 6XH
Tel: 08701 555 455
www.dh.gov.uk/publications
dh@prolog.uk.com

Your Weight Your Health Series
www.dh.gov.uk/publications

Eating Disorders Association
1st Floor
Wensum House
103 Prince of Wales Road
Norwich, Norfolk NR1 1DW
Tel: 01603 621414

Information and help on all aspects of eating disorders
www.edauk.com
helpmail@edauk.com
Adult helpline: 0845 634 141 (open 08.30–21.30 weekdays)
Youthline: 0845 634 7650 (open 16.00–18.30 weekdays, 13.00–16.30
Saturdays)

First Steps to Freedom
www.first-steps.org
Helpline: 08451202916 365 days a year 10.00–14.00
Offers confidential help, practical advice and support for phobias, including eating disorders.

Food Standards Agency
Aviation House
125 Kingsway
London WC2B 6NH
www.food.gov.uk

Healthy Schools
www.wiredforhealth.gov.uk
Information on healthy schools initiative

www.foodinschools.org
Information on school meals

MIND
National Association for Mental Health
Granta House
15–19 Broadway
Stratford, London E15 4BQ
www.mind.org.uk
Tel: 020 8519 2122
Fax: 020 8522 1725
contact@mind.org.uk
mindinfoline: 0845 766 0163
Offers fact sheets and booklets. Has a database of local groups, by post code.

The Royal College of Psychiatrists
www.rcpsych.ac.uk/info/eatdis.htm
An information site for eating disorders – includes leaflets, fact sheets, books and reports on eating disorders.

Chapter 8

Wound Management in General Practice

Joy Rudge

This chapter uses the example of wound management to relate some of the theoretical issues discussed within the book to practical care within general practice. These issues can be transferred to most clinical scenarios. Although the healing process has not changed, there have been advances in advances in wound management since the first edition, and these are discussed in some detail.

The principles of wound care relate to all wounds, regardless of size or position, and involve promoting healing within an optimum environment, using correct materials and methods of application.

Practice nurses, who are often the initial point of contact for wound management in primary care, must have evidence-based knowledge to make a skilled holistic assessment of both the patient and the wound to enable an appropriate cost-effective treatment plan to be devised.

The range of wounds encountered by the practice nurse will vary greatly, as will the autonomy for treatment allowed within individual general practices. Wound management is a dynamic area of healthcare with research leading to the development of new treatments. The following information should enable the reader to understand the rationale behind current wound management theories, assess the patient and choose an appropriate dressing/treatment. References that have not been updated since the 1st edition are still applicable.

Types of wound

A wound is an abnormal break in the skin, as a result of cell death or damage. Wounds are often categorised or classified, to enable professionals to share information and experiences knowing they are talking about similar wounds. Although classified in several ways, each wound is unique, and as such

The Informed Practice Nurse, Edwards, M. (2008), Chichester: Wiley.

Table 8.1   The UK Consensus classification of pressure sores (Reid & Morison 1994)

Stage	Findings
Stage 1	Discoloration of intact skin (light finger pressure applied to the intact skin does not alter the discoloration)
Stage 2	Partial thickness skin loss or damage involving epidermis and/or dermis
Stage 3	Full thickness skin loss involving damage to or necrosis of subcutaneous tissue but not extending to underlying bone, tendon or joint capsule
Stage 4	Full thickness skin loss with extensive destruction and tissue necrosis extending to underlying bone, tendon or joint capsules

deserves individual care. Wounds can also be categorised by the type of tissue within the wound:

- the wound is red and granulating
- the wound is starting to display signs of the formation of new pink epithelial tissue
- the wound is yellow and sloughing
- the wound contains black necrotic tissue
- the wound is green or infected.

These tissue types are discussed in more detail under wound assessment.

Wounds can also be classified by depth. This is a common way of describing pressure sores, several different scales existing for this. An example of this type of scale is the UK consensus classification of pressure sore severity (Stirling Scale) (Reid & Morison 1994), as shown in Table 8.1.

Although it is not usual to see pressure sores in the General Practitioner's surgery, anecdotally district nurses have referred mobile patients with post-operative sacral and heel pressure sores to the practice nurse for ongoing management. However, this type of classification by depth can be used or adapted to describe other wounds. Other methods of categorising wounds that can be used include by cause or by the stage of the healing process that the wound has reached.

The healing process

Wound healing is commonly classified as by primary, secondary or tertiary intention.

Primary intention healing should be achieved for all incised surgical wounds and primary sutured lacerations. Sutures, clips, adhesive glue or adhesive strips hold skin edges together. Healing should be rapid because there is no tissue loss and the skin edges are held together.

Secondary intention describes healing when skin edges are not brought together, and have to heal by contracting and filling up with granulation tissue before new epidermis can cover the wound. Examples of these wounds include leg ulcers, pressure damage or dirty surgical or traumatic injuries that may become infected if the skin edges are opposed and secured, open incisions, for example after draining abscesses when closure may encourage infection, and full thickness burns.

Tertiary intention is desirable if the wound such as a laceration has been contaminated, for example with animal bites. The wound is initially cleaned and left open; if there appears to be little risk of infection it may be closed in the normal way.

Wound healing is usually described in four physiological phases; inflammatory, destructive, proliferative and maturation phases. In reality this is a continuous process with the stages merging and overlapping.

Inflammatory stage 0–3 days

When tissue is injured or disrupted the body's immediate response is to re-establish haemostasis. Damaged cells and blood vessels release histamine, causing vasodilatation of the surrounding capillaries, which takes serous exudate and white cells to the area of damage (see Figure 8.1).

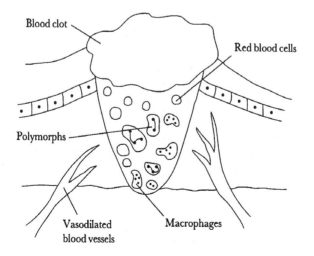

Figure 8.1 Inflammatory stage 0–3 days.

This increased blood flow and serous exudate causes local oedema, redness and heat resulting in an inflamed appearance. The coagulation system and platelets cause the blood to clot, preventing further bleeding or loss of body fluids. Injured vessels thrombose and red cells become entangled in a fibrin mesh, which begins to dry and becomes a scab. This is the body's natural defence to keep out microorganisms. Phagocytic white cells (polymorphs and macrophages) are attracted to the area to defend against bacteria, ingest debris and begin the process of repair. In a clean acute wound this stage lasts up to three days; if the wound is infected or necrotic tissue is present this stage is prolonged.

Destructive phase 1–6 days

This phase is illustrated in Figure 8.2. White cells line the walls of blood vessels and migrate through the walls, which are more porous, into surrounding tissue. Phagocytic cells break down devitalised necrotic tissue and the macrophages engulf and ingest bacteria and dead tissue. In addition, macrophages stimulate the development of new blood vessels and stimulate the formation and multiplication of fibroblasts, which in turn are responsible for the synthesis of collagen and other connective tissue. This stage normally lasts 1–6 days but white cell activity can be compromised in dry, exposed wounds.

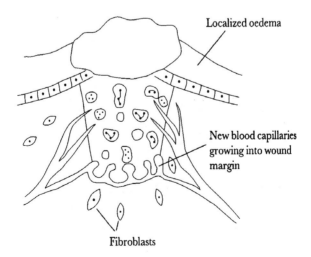

Figure 8.2 Destructive/migratory stage 1–6 days.

Proliferative phase 3–24 days

The fibroblasts continue to multiply, forming collagen fibrils which form a fibrous network (see Figure 8.3). This traps red blood cells, which go on to become new capillary loops. At this stage the tissue is very delicate having none of the organisation of normal tissue. This granulation tissue is so called because of its red granular appearance. As the collagen matures there is a rapid increase in tensile strength. Signs of inflammation subside and the process of contraction begins. In an open wound this stage may be prolonged because more collagen is needed to repair the tissue defect.

Maturation phase 24 days–1 year

As seen in Figure 8.4, when the wound has filled with granulation tissue, the collagen fibres pull in a wound causing it to contract and become smaller. This speeds up the healing process, as less collagen will be necessary to repair the defect. As the wound space decreases, vascularity also decreases, fibroblasts shrink and collagen fibres change the red granulation tissue to white avascular tissue as epithelium migrates inward.

Epithelial cells migrate over granulation tissue from the wound edge, sweat glands and the remnants of hair follicles until they meet with like cells from another area of the wound, sometimes forming islands in the wound centre. This process is slowed down if the wound is dry and is covered by a scab (or eschar). In this case they have to burrow under the dry scab. (See moist wound healing below.) Migrating cells lose their ability to divide, so epithelialisation depends on the ability of like cells to keep meeting. When the surface is covered with epithelial cells the epithelium thins. Hair follicles are not replaced. Wound maturation usually takes between 24 days and one year.

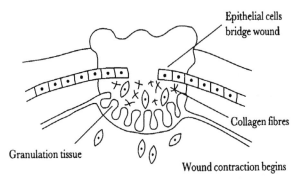

Figure 8.3   Proliferation/granulation stage 3–24 days.

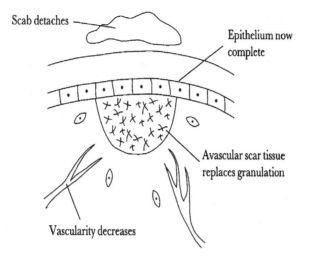

Scab detaches

Epithelium now complete

Avascular scar tissue replaces granulation

Vascularity decreases

Figure 8.4 Maturation stage 24 days–1 year.

Moist wound healing

Scab formation was thought to provide a mechanical barrier to infection and be the most appropriate treatment for wounds. Extensive research has shown that this is not the case, although many patients still cling to this traditional thought and challenge modern treatments.

Work on moist wound healing started in the early 1960s. The most quoted research in relation to this is the work of Winter (1962), who conducted a clinical trial using superficial wounds on pigs. The results showed that wounds covered with polythene epithelialized nearly twice as fast as those wounds allowed to dry out. Epithelial cells in the moist wounds could migrate more quickly through the wound exudate and did not need to traverse a scabbed area. This is supported by Dyson, Young & Pendle (1988) who showed that a moist wound moves through the inflammatory stage of healing more quickly than a dry wound and produces greater capillary growth.

It was initially thought that the moist environment might encourage greater bacterial growth and lead to a higher number of wound infections. Hutchinson and Lawrence (1991) disproved this view with studies that showed that the reverse was true and occluded wounds showed a lower rate of infection.

Since the late 1970s, manufacturing companies have been creating dressings that give a moist environment to speed wound healing. Modern products encourage wounds to heal faster and become infected less often. The comparatively high unit cost of some dressings becomes less relevant when viewed in relation to patient discomfort, patient and carer time, nursing time, greater use of other materials (for example, gloves, aprons, dressing packs) and antibiotics.

Wound assessment

Our medical colleagues are often grateful to delegate the responsibility of wound management to the nurse. In order for appropriate care to be given it is important that thorough assessment identifies a goal of treatment and clear management plan, with evaluation to check for progress or deterioration and patient concordance.

It is also important that this assessment and subsequent evaluations are clearly documented. Firstly, it allows evaluation to take place. Poor record keeping may result in an evaluation being vague and subjective, with reliance on comments such as 'looking better', or 'healing well', which tell us nothing about the state of the wound. This is perhaps even more important when more than one person is responsible for the patient's care. Secondly, records are of extreme importance in case of complaint or litigation. In legal terms if it is not recorded the care did not happen, so records must be timely, accurate and clear (see Chapter 1).

Activity 8.1

Review the records of a patient currently receiving wound care management. What do these records tell you about the wound appearance and history? Would you be happy to stand in court and defend your practice relying on the records you have made?

Although assessment may seem a lengthy process, time spent assessing a wound should lead to the selection of appropriate treatment, following discussion with the patient. This should optimise wound healing and lead to swifter resolution of care (see Chapter 2, time management). In the longer term the patient requires fewer episodes of care. Assessment details can be written into the patient notes or a purpose made chart can be completed and scanned into the patient records (see Figure 8.5). The following guidelines suggest areas to include.

Patient name ....   Position of wound ....

Type of wound ....   Duration of wound ....

Date							
Size of wound Max. width Max. length							
Type of tissue within wound e.g. slough, necrotic, granulation tissue							
Exudate Amount, colour?							
Odour None, some, offensive?							
Pain When, where, severity?							
Surrounding skin Erythema, wet/dry eczema							
Infection Suspected, swab taken, result?							
Treatment summary: Cleansing lotion Topical treatment of wound and surrounding skin Primary dressing Secondary dressing Fixed by							
Assessed by							

Figure 8.5 Example of a wound assessment form.

Wound type

Personal observation suggests that acute wounds such as lacerations, bites and post-operative wounds are usually clearly identified, but chronic wounds such as leg ulcers are generalised. It is important that the exact underlying causes identified. Is it a venous ulcer? Is it an arterial ulcer? Is it a malignancy? Did the wound start from trauma or a bite, in which case there may be no underlying disease.

The treatment for each wound type is different, and in the case of venous and arterial ulcers opposite, so without identification the chosen treatment may be incorrect. (Leg ulcers will be discussed in more detail below.)

Position of the wound

This should be clearly documented and may be aided by use of diagrams or photographs. The position of leg ulcers can also aid diagnosis.

Size of the wound

This should be recorded so that healing or deterioration can be noted. Both the nurse and the patient can be motivated if healing can be observed.

This also encourages patient concordance to continue with treatment not met with enthusiasm, such as compression therapy. The simplest way to record wound size is to take the maximum dimensions with a ruler (see Figure 8.6).

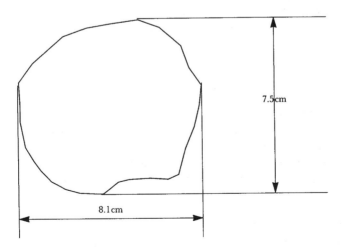

7.5 cm

8.1 cm

Figure 8.6 Measuring a wound.

A more accurate way is to trace the wound, using either purpose made charts (available from several dressing manufacturing companies), acetate sheets or the clear packaging in which many dressings come. The tracing can either be stored in the patient notes, or used as a template to draw round and add to notes. Consider whether or not the plastic is sterile. It is advisable to hold non-sterile materials slightly above the wound surface or to cleanse the surface touching the wound both before and after use with an alcohol wipe.

Photographs are the most accurate way to record size and appearance of large wounds. A Polaroid camera is useful to obtain instant pictures; this can be scanned into the patient records. Ideally digital photographs are downloaded directly into the patient records, thus preserving confidentiality. Personal cameras should not be used. Try to keep the background plain so that the patient's limb and wound stand out. It is also useful to attach a piece of tape on which the date and patient's initials are written; this helps identify photographs or checking chronological order.

The depth of the wound is more difficult to measure; using a sterile probe is probably the most accurate method. These are sometimes available from pharmaceutical companies, and are included with some ribbon dressing products.

History of the wound

It is worth asking how long the wound has been present, who up until now has being dressing it and what treatments have already been used. This will give some indication of any allergies or treatments that have previously failed. The wound may be a recurrence of a leg ulcer (particularly venous) and the treatment of previous episodes of ulceration may be relevant.

Surrounding skin

It is important to assess the surrounding skin. Any redness or erythema may indicate infection. If the patient has fragile skin, perhaps caused by medication such as long-term steroid use, it may be inappropriate to apply an adhesive dressing. Leg ulcers may be surrounded by varicose eczema that requires an emollient, or by contact dermatitis from previous treatments, which may require a short cause of a topical steroid cream.

Tissue within the wound

The state of the tissue within the wound will help to identify the goal of treatment and in many ways identify an appropriate treatment. There may be more than one type of tissue within the wound, in which case an estimate of the percentage of each type should be made, for example 70% granulation and 30% slough.

The wound may contain *black* or *necrotic tissue*, which is the result of tissue death secondary to ischaemia. It may be soft and spongy or form a hard eschar over the surface of the wound. This will always delay healing and increases the chances of wound infection. The aim of treatment is debridement by using an appropriate dressing or, if necessary, a surgical opinion on sharp debridement can be sought.

The *yellow* or *sloughy tissue* formed in many chronic wounds is made up of dead cells and serous exudate. This needs to be removed to optimise healing and is a similar process to debridement. It is important not to mistake exposed tendons or epithelial islands for slough as they may have a similar appearance.

Red or *granulating* wounds have fragile, easily damaged new tissue forming. The aim of treatment is to protect the tissue and provide a moist environment to optimise healing. Particular care should be taken during dressing changes. The selected dressing should not adhere to the surface of the wound and cause trauma when removed.

Pink or *epithelial tissue* is the new layer of epidermis that covers the wound once it has filled with granulation tissue. Epithelial cells that migrate from the wound margins sometimes meet to form clusters or islands on the wound surface. A moist environment aids movement of these cells, so the chosen dressing should again provide this environment and protect the wound surface.

Infected tissue within the wound often has a *greenish* appearance. Routine wound swabbing is inappropriate for diagnosis of infection and is an unnecessary cost. It is important to understand that wounds may have transient organisms present that swab results detect in small numbers. These organisms are often the usual skin flora and are not usually regarded as pathogenic.

Many chronic wounds become colonised by a variety of bacteria that may be potentially pathogenic. *Colonisation* refers to organisms that have multiplied and are often present in high numbers but infection is not inevitable and many colonised wounds heal without problem. These microorganisms can however be dispersed during dressing changes and measures should be taken to limit this (see Chapter 3).

Some wounds quickly progress from colonisation to infection. Others move from being colonised to a critically colonised state and remain in this state as an indolent wound that is not visibly deteriorating. Critical colonisation can be suspected if the wound fails to respond to appropriate care, pain levels increase (without obvious cellulitis), slough fails to lift when treated

---

Box 8.1   Criteria that may indicate infection

- delayed healing
- discoloration
- friable granulation tissue that bleeds easily
- unexpected tenderness
- pocketing at the base of the wound
- bridging of soft tissue and epithelium
- wound breakdown.

---

appropriately, slough returns quickly after rapid debridement (for example, surgical/larval) or odour levels increase (White 2003).

Wound infection occurs when colonising bacteria reach sufficient numbers to cause distinct clinical signs. These include erythema, oedema, increased exudate, offensive odour, pain and pyrexia. If a wound exhibits one or more of these signs it is appropriate to take a wound swab. Immunocompromised or diabetic patients may fail to show signs of inflammation or clinical infection and may require a wound swab to be taken if the wound is failing to respond to treatment, even if the usual clinical signs are not present. Cooper and Lawrence (1996) recommended gentle irrigation of the wound with normal saline, and swabbing in a zigzag motion over the entire wound surface while slowly rotating the swab.

If wounds fail to respond to treatment it is worth considering seven other criteria that may indicate infection (Box 8.1).

The treatment of infection should be by systemic antibiotics. Topical antibacterial creams can lead to the growth of resistant organisms, and are not recommended (Morgan 1987) although products containing antimicrobials may be useful (Molan 2001; Thomas 2004). See sections on honey and silver dressings.

Pain

The patient's level of pain should be assessed and treated with appropriate analgesia. Other factors to consider are:

- is the pain ischaemic? (if the leg ulcer is arterial, a vascular opinion may be appropriate – see below)
- is the wound infected?

- is the dressing causing pain by either drying and adhering to the wound surface, or causing an allergic reaction?
- is the wound painful at dressing change because the dressing is being removed inappropriately?

Wound odour

Wound odour often occurs in heavily infected or fungating wounds and can be very distressing for the patient. Personal experience shows that this may be one reason a patient has sought treatment. Some dressings may cause odour when they interact with wound exudate; pre-warn the patient if this is expected to happen either at dressing change or if the dressing leaks.

Charcoal dressings should be used to combat odour if available. Oral or topical metronidazole may reduce odour (Newman, Allwood & Oakes 1989), and aromatherapy oils may be applied to the outer dressing to mask the odour, although this may not be successful.

General assessment of the patient – factors affecting healing

During the assessment it is important to look at the patient holistically. Many factors influence wound healing. Some of these are listed in Box 8.2. If these are not addressed, healing will be delayed or may even fail to take place. Not all factors can be treated but, if highlighted, at least the nurse can gain an understanding of why healing is slow.

Box 8.2   Factors affecting wound healing

- age
- concurrent disease
- nutritional status
- drugs
- smoking
- excessive alcohol consumption
- infection
- non-concordance of treatment by patient.

Age

As people age their metabolic processes slow down, which prolongs tissue repair. Wound infection may also be more common as immune competence becomes less specific and inflammation less effective (David 1986). The elderly are more likely to have chronic concurrent illness that requires a range of treatments that may delay healing.

Concurrent disease

Diabetes has long been associated with poor wound healing so it is important to control blood sugar levels if wound healing is to be achieved. Diabetics are also more susceptible to wound infection.

Cardiovascular and pulmonary disease may delay wound healing because transport of oxygen to the wound site may be inadequate, and oxygen is essential for wound healing.

Uraemia increases the risk of wound dehiscence due to a reduction in collagen deposition. Granulation may also be delayed.

Thyroid or pituitary deficiency may delay healing as a result of slowed metabolic rates. Cushing's syndrome treated with steroids will also delay healing.

Nutritional status

Both obesity and malnourishment inhibit wound healing. Gross obesity is likely to make the patient less mobile, thus leading to venous stasis. Adipose tissue is also poorly oxygenated. Advice from a community dietician may be necessary for some patients.

Poor nutrition and malnourishment adversely affect wound healing in many ways. The links between nutrients and healing are shown in Table 8.2.

Table 8.2 Important nutrients in wound healing

Nutrient	Role in wound healing
Protein	Repair and replacement of tissue
	Energy
Carbohydrate	Energy
	Spares protein for wound healing
Vitamin C	Collagen synthesis
	Immunity
Vitamin B12	Protein synthesis
Zinc	Tissue repair
	Protein synthesis
Iron	Haemoglobin production

It should be remembered that injury might also lead to a patient's energy demands being higher than usual, and that protein is also lost in wound exudate.

If a patient is unable to maintain a good nutritional status, dietary supplements may be necessary, either in the form of tablets (for example, zinc supplements or multivitamins); by injection (for example, hydroxycobalamin or iron); or as meal replacements or supplements. This should be discussed with the dietician and/or medical practitioner.

Drug therapy

Drugs taken therapeutically for other conditions may inhibit wound healing:

- *Anti-inflammatory* drugs, both steroidal and non-steroidal, will delay wound healing. These drugs are designed to suppress inflammation, which is essential for tissue repair.
- *Immunosupressive* drugs inhibit white cell activity and thus delay the clearance of wound debris. Patients on these drugs are at a high risk of developing a wound infection and may require prophylactic antimicrobial therapy and careful monitoring. Thought needs to be given to timing appointments for these patients in order to reduce the risks of cross-infection (see Chapter 2, Management, and Chapter 3, Infection control).
- *Cytotoxic* drugs arrest cell division and also reduce protein production. This is true for both malignant cells and those vital for tissue repair.

Smoking

Smoking alters platelet function leading to a higher risk of blood clots blocking smaller vessels. Smokers also have reduced haemoglobin function (David 1986), resulting in less haemoglobin being available for oxygen transport, which adversely affects wound healing. The risk of arterial disease is increased, which may cause tissue ischaemia and necrosis.

Alcohol

Patients who are heavy drinkers may have liver disease, which can result in a reduction in the number of platelets and clotting functions. They may also have a lower resistance to infection. Gastritis and diarrhoea may also predispose to malnourishment through malabsorption and anaemia caused by blood loss.

Non-concordance

Most nurses will have encountered patients who interfere with their dress-ings, either because they are not happy with the treatment plan, find the dressings uncomfortable or are simply confused. The importance of involv-ing patients in their treatment cannot be overstated (see Chapter 1).

Wound cleansing

Cleansing wounds by swabbing with cotton wool or gauze results in the materials shedding fibres into the wound, which may act as a focus for infec-tion (Draper 1985). Vigorous swabbing may also damage healthy tissue. Irrigation is therefore generally the preferred method, but care should be taken to prevent splash back and a visor worn if appropriate.

Which wounds will benefit from cleansing?

Traumatic wounds that contain particles of dirt or other matter will benefit from vigorous irrigation (Lawrence 1997). Wounds may also benefit from cleansing to remove gross exudate, the remains of previous topical applica-tions or crusting (Lawrence 1997; Miller & Dyson 1996). Research suggests that cleansing to remove bacteria is ineffective (Miller & Dyson 1996); bac-teria are not removed, but merely redistributed around the wound surface. Cleansing is only appropriate to remove debris or old dressing material. Explain the reasons for not cleansing to the patient to avoid any misunder-standings, because most patients think cleansing is essential.

What fluid should be used for wound cleansing?

The most frequently used fluids are tap water, sterile saline or antiseptics.

Antiseptics

There is little evidence to suggest that use of antiseptics reduces the bacterial content of wounds, and wounds do not need to be sterile to heal. Miller and Dyson (1996) list some of the criticisms levied against antiseptics:

- antiseptics do not come into contact with bacteria long enough to kill them during normal wound cleansing
- bacteria may become resistant to antiseptics and those antiseptics con-taining cetrimide or chlorehexidine may grow bacteria under certain conditions

- the frequent use of antiseptics may contribute towards bacterial resistance to antibiotics, although there is no proven link
- antiseptics adversely affect blood flow in the healing wound
- antiseptics are inactivated by organic matter such as pus and wound exudates.

If an antiseptic is to be used the following are suggested by Lawrence (1997) as the safer options:

- Chlorhexidine solutions – this is a good skin and hard surface disinfectant and shows low toxicity to living tissue in animal models.
- Povidone iodine – iodine kills bacteria rapidly, possibly within a few seconds, but can impair the micro-circulation in animals. Beware of iodine sensitivity.

Tap water

One study conducted with tap water found that there was less infection in wounds cleansed with tap water and no bacteria were transferred to the wound (Angeras, Brandberg, Falk & Seeman 1991). However, some cell damage may occur as a result of lowered osmotic pressure, which may result in pain (Lawrence 1997).

Sterile normal saline

Saline in a 0.9% solution has similar osmotic pressures to that found in the tissue in mammals. This reinforces the fact that saline baths are inappropriate because the concentrations vary widely. Saline is currently favoured as the treatment of choice, minimising the risk of tissue damage and pain. This should be used as warm solution.

The ideal dressing

The criteria for the ideal dressing suggested by Morgan (1987) have not been challenged, and still apply in 2008. The most important will be discussed and implications for nursing practice highlighted.

The dressing should provide a moist environment

A primary factor in optimising healing is that the dressing should provide a moist environment (see above). All of the modern occlusive dressings should provide this type of environment.

Nursing implication: No dry dressings should be used on open wounds because these will allow the area to dry out and thus impede healing.

The wound should be kept free from excess exudates

Although the wound needs to be kept moist it must not be wet. This causes the surrounding skin to become soggy and macerated and may lead to further tissue breakdown.

Nursing implication: A dressing should be selected that provides the correct amount of absorbency. All dressings are designed with particular types of wound in mind; for example, alginates are designed for highly exuding wounds, and vapour-permeable films for wounds with very little exudate. This is an important criterion in dressing selection.

The dressing should provide thermal insulation

Wound healing is optimised when wounds are kept at body temperature. If the temperature of the wound drops, mitotic activity slows down, thus reducing wound healing. A drop in wound temperature will also disrupt leukocytic activity and oxyhaemaglobin dissociation (Miller & Dyson 1996; Thomas 1990).

Nursing implication: Lock (1980) and Myers (1982) found that after cleansing it could take a wound up to 40 minutes to regain body temperature and a further three hours for mitotic activity to return to normal. Thus it is advisable to warm saline prior to wound cleansing, to keep wounds exposed for as short a time as possible, to try not to disturb wounds unnecessarily and to consider the type of material being used. For example, cotton gauze will keep a wound at around 27°C whereas a hydrocolloid or foam dressing will increase that to 35°C (Thomas 1990).

The dressing should be impermeable to microorganisms

This should work in both directions. While microorganisms should be kept away from wounds, it is also undesirable to have microorganisms from a wound spreading to the environment.

Nursing implication: Any non-adhesive dressing should be taped like a 'picture frame' if surrounding skin is in good condition, or bandaged to cover the dressing completely. If 'strike through' occurs, a warm wet passage for microorganisms is created, and secondary padding should be applied or the wound redressed. Patients should be advised to return to the surgery if strike through occurs.

The dressing should be free from particulate contaminants

Modern dressings are designed to high standards and will not shed fibres or contaminants onto the wound surface. However, traditional gauze, lint or cotton wool may shed fibres that can serve as a focus for infection.

Nursing implication: No dry dressings that shed fibres should be applied directly onto an open wound.

The dressing should not cause trauma to the wound

If the chosen dressing adheres to the wound, trauma and pain may occur on dressing removal. Modern dressings provide the ideal healing environment and are free from materials that adhere.

Nursing implication: Traditional dressings such as cotton gauze and paraffin gauze should not be used on open wounds. The wound exudate becomes incorporated into the gauze and dries out, adhering to the tissue below. The top layer of granulation tissue is removed with the dressing. Paraffin gauze leaves a criss-cross pattern where new granulation tissue has grown through the mesh, illustrating the pattern quite graphically.

The dressing should allow gaseous exchange

This is a complex issue. It has been noted that angiogenisis (formation of new blood vessels) in granulating wounds takes place rapidly in the hypoxic environment of occlusive dressings such as hydrocolloids (Cherry & Ryan 1985). However, when a wound begins to show signs of new epidermis forming this appears more effective in a more oxygen rich environment (Silver 1985).

Nursing implication: It may be appropriate to use an occlusive dressing when a wound needs to granulate but better to switch to an oxygen permeable dressing (for example, a foam dressing) to encourage granulation.

The dressing should be available

Is the dressing available to community nurses? Can it be prescribed? If not how will you access it?

Nursing implication: It is illegal to order one item from the pharmacist and exchange this for something of the same value. Even though it is done with the patient's interest at heart this action constitutes fraud; if prosecuted the nurse could face a fine, imprisonment and dismissal.

At the time of writing no one dressing meets all these criteria. It is therefore important to assess the wound thoroughly, decide on a treatment goal and select the most appropriate dressing from those available.

Dressing types

Many types of wound dressing are available, and it can be difficult to choose the one most appropriate to the wound. This section attempts to place the dressings into broad categories with some suggestions for their appropriate use. The dressings mentioned are not the only ones available and for further information it would be appropriate to refer to a text such as *Mimms for Nurses* (2006), which is updated regularly. General practices often use a locality wound management formulary for ease and cost-effective prescribing

For information about methods of application, time between dressing changes, removal and contra-indications see manufacturers' instructions. Only dressings available on the drug tariff are discussed below.

Alginate dressings

These dressings are made from seaweed, which contains large quantities of alginate. They are highly absorbent so should not be used on wounds with very little exudate because they will adhere to the wound surface. Some clinicians wet the dressing with saline but this seems pointless as the dressing is designed to be highly absorbent.

Alginates form a gel on contact with wound exudate, giving a moist environment while absorbing excess fluid. They may be used on flat wounds and also to pack cavity wounds. A secondary dressing is required.

Examples of alginates are Kaltostat (Convatec), Seasorb Soft (Coloplast), Sorbsan and Sorbsan Plus (Unomedical) and Tegagel (3M).

Bead dressings

Polysaccharide beads are indicated for wet sloughy wounds and should not be used on clean or dry wounds. The beads are extremely hydrophilic and will cause pain if the wound is too dry. Iodosorb and Iodoflex (Smith and Nephew) both contain iodine and have been used with some success on wounds with superficial infection or superficial wounds contaminated with MRSA. All require a secondary dressing.

Foam dressings (including hydropolymer and hydrocellular dressings)

Foam dressings are generally highly absorbent and create a moist environment for wound healing; they can be used on a wide variety of wounds. They are available without adhesive, which is useful if the surrounding skin is damaged or fragile, or as adhesive dressings and can be used on their own or as a secondary dressing, e.g. with hydogels.

Non-adhesive foams include Allevyn (Smith and Nephew), Lyofoam and Lyofoam Extra (Molnlycke). Lyofoam is also useful for resolving over-granulation. Adhesive foams include Allevyn Adhesive (Smith and Nephew), Combiderm (Convatec), and Tielle (Johnson and Johnson).

Hydrogels

Amorphous gels have a high water content. They are very useful for debriding or desloughing wounds by rehydrating the dead tissue, thus allowing the body to shed this tissue by autolysis. Gels are designed for use on sloughy or necrotic wounds with low to medium exudate, but can also be used on flat wounds and to fill cavities. They are also reported to reduce pain at the wound site (Morgan 1994). They require a secondary dressing such a non-adherent dressing, padding and a bandage to secure. Examples of hydrogels are Intrasite gel (Smith and Nephew) and Nugel (Johnson and Johnson).

Hydrocolloid dressings

Hydrocolloid dressings made from combinations of synthetic polymers are one of the oldest of the 'modern' products and are used in many situations. They are waterproof, adhesive, interactive dressings that form a gel on contact with wound exudate. This may have a slight odour that is normal. Hydrocolloids can aid desloughing and can be used on light to medium exuding wounds. Their occlusive nature gives a hypoxic environment, which stimulates angiogenisis (Cherry & Ryan 1985) and the moist environment gives pain relief by keeping nerve endings moist (Morgan 1994).

Examples of hydrocolloids are Comfeel (Coloplast), Granuflex (Convatec) and Tegasorb (3M). Extra thin versions are also available as Comfeel Transparent (Coloplast) and Duoderm (Convatec). All the hydrocolloids can be used alone or as a secondary dressing (check manufacturers' recommendations).

Hydrocolloid gel dressings

Granugel (Convatec) is a gel that contains hydrocolloid for desloughing and debriding wounds, and can also be applied to clean wounds. It requires a secondary dressing such as Granuflex.

Vapour-permeable film dressings

These were the first type of modern dressings to be produced. Waterproof adhesive films create a moist environment but have no fluid handling capabilities. They can be used on superficial wounds with minimal exudate, prophylactically (for example, to reduce shearing forces), on wounds healing by primary intention or as secondary dressings securing or protecting other products, such as adhesive strips.

Examples of film dressings are Bioclusive (Johnson and Johnson), Opsite flexigrid (Smith and Nephew) and Tegaderm (3M).

Protease inhibitors

A new generation of products have been designed to react bioactively with chronic wounds (Stewart 2002).

Promogran matrix (Johnson and Johnson) is a topically applied therapy that is a freeze-dried matrix made up of collagen and oxidised regenerated cellulose. It is recommended for use on all types of chronic wounds, such as pressure sores and leg ulcers, which are free from necrotic tissue and signs of infection. A secondary dressing is required to maintain a moist wound-healing environment. This product binds and inactivates proteases that have been shown to become excessive in chronic wounds and impede the healing process and protects naturally occurring growth factors from these proteases (Stewart 2002).

Promagran Prisma matrix is a similar product but contains silver so can be used in the presence of signs of infection.

Cadesorb (Smith and Nephew) has been designed to reduce protease activity in chronic wounds by reducing the wound pH. It is available as an ointment and requires a secondary dressing.

Larval therapy

Larval, or maggot, therapy is used for the eradication of necrotic and infected tissue (Thomas, Jones & Andrews 1998). The use of certain species of larvae in wound healing has been recognised for centuries. The larvae of the *Lucilia sericata*, or green bottle, are used in wound management. The secretion of proteolytic enzymes from larval salivary and intestinal glands breaks down and liquefies necrotic tissue, which is then sucked up and digested. Larval therapy can be used on many types of necrotic or infected wounds including:

- leg ulcers (Jones & Champion 1998; Sherman 1998)
- pressure sores (Thomas et al. 1998)
- infected surgical and traumatic wounds (Evans 1997; Sherman 1998)
- MRSA infected wounds (Thomas & Jones 2005).

Larval therapy is contraindicated in the following wounds: those containing hard black eschar – a hydrogel is first applied to rehydrate the tissue, but this should be thoroughly washed off prior to application of larvae as pro-pylene glycol has been found to have adverse effects on larvae viability and growth (Thomas & Jones 2005); and fistula or wounds that might connect to vital organs.

Caution is needed with the following wounds: near exposed blood vessels – monitor for blood loss (Thomas et al 1999); and with ischaemic leg ulcers – the therapy may increase wound pain as a result of a change in the wound pH (Thomas, Andrews, Hay & Bourgoise 1999).

Sterile larvae are now available on prescription. There are approximately 200 larvae per pot, which are delivered in clear plastic containers with a filter to allow larvae to breathe and a moist swab to prevent them drying out. There is also a medical grade nylon mesh to retain the larvae after applica-tion and a sterile solution of sodium chloride (normal saline). The number of pots required will depend on wound size and percentage of necrotic tissue. A larvae calculator is available from the supplier STML healthcare – Tel: 01656 752820. There is no need to count larvae on application or removal.

Application of larvae

The wound is surrounded by a hydrocolloid dressing, leaving the wound exposed (like a picture frame). Larvae are flushed on to the net with the saline. Invert the net containing the larvae on to the wound; secure the net to the hydrocolloid using water resistant adhesive tape. Place a swab moist-ened with saline over the outer surface of the net; apply padding and ban-dages as required (Biosurgical Research Unit 2003).

Larvae are left in place for up to three days. To remove, peel back the hydrocolloid and the rest of the dressing system including the larvae will follow. Dispose of larvae in two sealed yellow bags. Further larvae may be applied, or a conventional dressing used, dependent on the state of the wound. Readers are recommended to liase with community colleagues with experience of larval therapy before attempting application.

Note: LarvE net boots and sleeves are available for difficult areas such as feet. Zinc paste bandage is an alternative to hydrocolloid if the patient has a known sensitivity to hydrocolloids or has fragile skin.

Silver dressings

The development of antibiotics in the twentieth century led to the decline of many former remedies but the emergence of antibiotic resistant strains of pathogens, particularly meticillin-resistant *Staphlococcus aureus* (MRSA) (see Chapter 3), has led to the need to find alternative treatments (Cooper 2004, Thomas 2004). The antimicrobial property of silver has been used medicinally since the nineteenth century, while the ancient Greek and Roman civilizations are thought to have used silver coins to make water drinkable (White 2003).

There are now a number of silver dressings available, which slowly release a small steady amount of ionic silver ions over a period of time. This slow release decreases the risk of silver toxicity and helps to ensure a decreased bacterial level (Cutting 2003).

Silver dressings are indicated in the following cases:

- Wound infection: although antibiotics are indicated in overt wound infection where the classical signs are evident (Cooper 2004)
- As an intervention to prevent the development of systemic infection in a critically colonised wound: in this instance systemic antibiotics are not always appropriate and topical antimicrobial treatments may be more suitable (Cooper 2004)
- In chronic wounds: reduction of certain microbial species, such as anaerobic bacteria in order to limit undesirable odours is justified (Forrest 1982)
- Prophylactic use may prevent the development of infections, thus minimising antibiotic use in patients with a history of repeated wound infections (Cooper 2004).

Although reports of resistance are limited, misuse and abuse of silver must be avoided. Silver should only be used for short periods of time, for example 2–3 weeks (Morris 2006).

Silver sulphadiazine has also been linked to argyria (the deposition of silver in the skin) when used on large areas of for a prolonged time (British National Formulary 2007). Most silver dressings are more expensive than 'plain' versions; therefore their use should be appropriate and not routine.

Examples of silver dressings are Acticoat (Smith and Nephew), Aquacel Ag (Convatec) and Urgotul SSD (Urgo).

Dressings containing honey

Honey is another ancient treatment for infected wounds, which has recently been 'rediscovered' (Molan 2001). It is reported to have an inhibitory effect on around 60 species of bacteria (including MRSA) and on some fungal infections and can be used prophylactically on patients susceptible to MRSA or other wound infections. Honey dressings also facilitate autolytic debridement and reduce malodour.

Available honey dressings include Medihoney (Medihoney) and Mesitran (Molnlycke).

Cost effectiveness

The cost effectiveness of treatments must be considered when selecting products. While some newer products may have a higher unit cost than more traditional methods, the overall cost may be reduced if they enhance wound healing (Stewart 2002). It is important to select a product that is suitable for the wound and which has been shown to be effective. Using only one product on a wound rather than multiple primary treatments together in layers can reduce costs.

Management of minor traumatic wounds

Patients present in general practice with a variety of minor injuries. It is important that where there is any doubt about underlying damage the patient is advised to attend casualty.

Cleaning

Wounds that have been caused accidentally are likely to be contaminated with dirt or bacteria. In addition to treating the wound the patient will need advice about tetanus cover and any antibiotic therapy that may be required, for example following a dog bite. Wounds should be thoroughly irrigated with warmed normal saline or tap water to remove as much dirt and contamination as possible. Grazes often contain grit and grime, which must be removed to avoid a tattooing effect when the graze has healed. It is important to ensure no fragments, such as glass or metal, remain in the wound. The patient should be advised to attend casualty for an X-ray and removal of glass or metal fragments.

Closure

Once clean, it is important to decide whether it is possible to close the wound. Larger wounds, wounds to the face or those over a joint may require suturing. Smaller lacerations may be held together with reinforced adhesive strips. The skin edges should be brought together as close as possible. Ensure the skin is dry and place the first tape in the centre of the wound. Use further closures to oppose the sides of the wound, and then place further ones in any gaps to give a neat finish. Cover with a non-adherent dressing and remove in 5–7 days.

Surgical glue can be useful in managing some straight wounds, especially in children and for scalp wounds. It is not suitable for areas with tension, such as over a joint. Application is less traumatic for the child who will not require local anaesthetic or sutures, and it also reduces medical and nursing time. Refer to the manufacturer's instructions for application.

Tying the hairs from either side of the wound prevents shaving the area and gives a neat scar, and may close small scalp wounds, although this is difficult with short hair.

Pretibial lacerations are common in the elderly, who have very fragile skin, so great care must be taken to ensure that no further skin tears are made. A skin flap may be taped back into place, but is often too thin to be viable as it has a poor blood supply to the superficial tissue. In this case trimming the flap is an option, allowing the wound to heal by secondary intention. Often a simple dressing such as Inadine, a nonadherent dressing and a retention banadage is the most appropriate management for this type of wound. A patient who has vascular changes, with a poor arterial blood supply may have delayed wound healing, while poor venous circulation may result in a venous ulcer.

Burns

Small burns and scalds are commonly seen in general practice. Any burn of significant size, of full thickness, over a joint or on the face should be referred to casualty. Initial treatment is to cool the surface of the burn or scald with cool water for a minimum of 10 minutes, or until it no longer hurts. Blisters should be left intact, as microorganisms cannot enter intact skin. Where blisters have ruptured, wound treatment will depend on the tissue state. The wound can be initially treated with Flamazine (silver sulphadiazine), paraffin gauze or Mepitel, a nonadherent dressing and padding, review after one day and assess for treatment as wound needs dictate.

Management of post-operative wounds

Surgical wounds are usually closed with sutures or clips, which are left in place for between 5–14 days depending on the type of surgery, and the depth of the wound they are closing.

Studies have shown that after 24 hours the skin will have formed a natural barrier at the suture or clip line, which means a dressing may be unnecessary (Chrintz 1989). Patients require dressings if there is any leakage from the suture line or as a protection to the wound from friction by clothing. Certain areas, such as the groin following varicose vein surgery, may require a light dressing to absorb any perspiration and reduce friction. Dressings such as Opsite Plus or Mepore Ultra have an absorbent pad and are shower proof. They are comfortable and can be left in place until suture removal. Once sutures or clips have been removed a dressing should not be necessary unless the wound continues to exude from any areas along the suture line.

Pilonidal sinus wounds can require daily dressings for several weeks. Patients should be advised (and encouraged) to have a shower before attending the practice. Options for packing the sinus include Sorbsan ribbon, Aquacel and Intrasite comfortable, depending on the level of exudate. Dressing type will change with the stage of wound healing.

Management of leg ulcers

Studies showed that between 65% and 85% of leg ulceration were managed exclusively by the primary healthcare team (Kendrick, Lucker, Cullum & Roe 1994). In 2008 management may be exclusively by the practice nurse, or in a shared clinic with district nursing colleagues. A leg ulcer can be defined as an area of discontinuity of the epidermis and dermis on the lower leg persisting for four weeks or more, excluding ulcers confined to the foot.

Causes of leg ulceration

Minor trauma is often the immediate cause of the ulcer but underlying pathology leads to ulcer development. The most common pathology is venous disease, but a significant number arise from other pathologies. It is important to determine the underlying cause to ensure correct management of the ulcer.

Box 8.3   Causes of leg ulceration

- Neuropathy – often associated with diabetes mellitus
- Malignancy – basal cell carcinoma, squamous cell carcinoma or melanoma
- Infections – tuberculosis, deep fungal infections, leprosy, syphilis; these are rare in the UK but should be considered particularly if the patient has been travelling or living in the tropics
- Lymphoedema – usually only associated with ulceration following cellulitis of if venous disease is also present
- Metabolic disorders – e.g. Pyoderma gangrenosum
- Blood disorders – e.g. sickle cell disease, thalassaemia
- Self inflicted ulcers
- Iatrogenic – these can be caused by ill-fitting plaster casts or badly applied bandages being used to treat existing ulcers

---

Common causes

1. Approximately 70% of ulcers are the result of venous disease, usually due to incompetent valves in the deep and perforating veins.
2. Around 10–15% arise from arterial disease when there is atherosclerotic occlusion of the large vessels or arteritis of small vessels. These changes lead to tissue ischaemia. Diabetes mellitus and rheumatoid arthritis can also cause changes to the smaller distal arteries. In addition, Raynaud's disease also affects the arterial circulation.
3. Approximately 10% of patients will have both venous and arterial disease, and their ulcers will be of mixed aetiology).

Other causes

Around 2–5% of patients develop ulcers due to other causes. Although rare these should be kept in mind (see Box 8.3).

Assessment

Successful treatment of leg ulcers requires thorough assessment and diagnosis of the underlying pathology. This should include assessment of the patient's general condition (Box 8.4), ulcer related history, clinical investigations and examination of the ulcer itself. Patient assessment and wound assessment have been discussed in some detail earlier in the chapter but an overview and issues specific to leg ulcers will be given here.

Box 8.4   Assessment of the patient's general condition

This should include:

- Age
- Sex
- Family history – there may be predisposing factors to leg ulcer development
- Occupational history – venous leg ulcers are often associated with occupations involving prolonged standing
- Mobility – reduced mobility contributes to ulcer development and poor healing
- Diet – poor nutritional status may delay healing
- Obesity – may contribute to ulcer development and poor healing
- Smoking habits – smoking may contribute to poor healing and circulatory disease
- General living conditions
- Psychological status – this is important in determining a patient's participation in care and their concordance with treatment

---

Ulcer related history

The assessment of a patient presenting with either a first or a recurrent leg ulcer should include a detailed history of the onset of the problem. A summary of medical histories that may be indicative of venous or arterial disease is shown in Box 8.5.

Ulcer specific history

This should include a history of any previous ulceration, with its duration, the treatments used and any known allergies to dressings. A history of the current episode of ulceration should also be documented.

Clinical investigations

Some routine investigations can aid the diagnosis of the leg ulcer or help in its management. Other investigations are only necessary in a few cases and include weight and tissue biopsy. These are summarised in Table 8.3.

Vascular assessment

The simplest form of vascular assessment is to palpate the dorsalis pedis and posterior tibial foot pulses, although the presence of oedema may make these

---

Box 8.5   Relevant medical history

A medical history of patients with *venous* disease may include any of the following:

- varicose veins – either treated or untreated
- deep vein thrombosis
- phlebitis of the affected leg
- suspected deep vein thrombosis, e.g. swollen leg following surgery, pregnancy or trauma
- surgery on affected leg
- trauma to affected leg such as a fracture
- history of pulmonary embolism.

A medical history suggestive of *arterial* involvement may include:

- hypertension myocardial infarction
- angina
- transient ischaemic attacks
- diabetes mellitus
- rheumatoid arthritis
- cerebrovascular accident.
- arterial surgery
- intermittent claudication
- peripheral vascular disease.

Table 8.3 Clinical investigations

Investigation	Rationale
Blood pressure measurement	To detect hypertension
Urinalysis/fasting sugar	To detect diabetes
Full blood count	To identify anaemia
Wound swab	If clinical signs of infection are present, to determine antibiotic sensitivity
Tissue biopsy	If malignancy is suspected
Weight	Dietary advice and weight reduction to aid healing

difficult to feel. It should, however, be noted that the dorsalis pedis pulse is congenitally absent in up to 12% of people (Barnhorst & Barner 1968). A more accurate way to ascertain the condition of the arterial circulation is to measure the ankle brachial pressure index (ABPI) using Doppler ultrasound. ABPI determines the ratio of the ankle to the brachial systolic pressure with the aid of a battery-operated handheld Doppler. Doppler readings should be undertaken when the patient first presents with an episode of ulceration, if the ulcer is deteriorating or when the ulcer is refractory to treatment after three months, and at regular six monthly intervals during treatment. Only a nurse who has received training and practised under supervision should do this. Refer to your district nursing colleagues if you are not trained in this procedure.

Examination of the legs and skin

The patient should have both legs thoroughly examined, whether ulcerated or not. Box 8.6 summarises the clinical signs and symptoms of both venous and arterial disease.

Box 8.6   Signs of venous and arterial disease

Signs of venous disease may include:

- varicose veins
- lipodermatosclerosis (hardening of the dermis and underlying sub-cutaneous fat.)
- stasis eczema
- ankle flare (the appearance of many dilated intradermal venules over the medial aspect of the ankle)
- staining of the skin due to breakdown products of haemoglobin from extravasted red blood cells
- atrophe blanche (areas of white skin with tiny red spots that are dilated capillary loops).

Signs of arterial disease may include:

- cold legs and feet in a warm environment
- pale or blue feet when raised
- feet dusky pink when dependent
- shiny hairless leg
- gangrenous toes
- absent foot pulses
- trophic changes to nails
- poor tissue perfusion, if direct pressure is applied to the nail bed return to normal colour takes longer than three seconds

---

Table 8.4   Common differences in the appearance of venous and arterial ulcers

Venous ulcers
Site: often near the medial or lateral malleolus Depth and shape: usually shallow with a poorly defined edge Pain: the pain of venous ulceration is often associated with oedema, from local infections or cellulitis. Pain can be relieved by support bandages and elevation Development: usually slow unless infected
Arterial ulcers
Site: often on the foot or lateral aspect of the leg but may occur anywhere including the malleolar areas Depth and shape: often deep with a punched out appearance, often irregular shapes or multiple small areas Pain: invariably painful, often the pain is made worse by elevation or exercise. Patient may report hanging the legs out of bed to relieve pain Development: often rapid

Oedema may be present with either venous or arterial disease, but its presence should be noted and other possible causes investigated and eliminated.

Examination of the ulcer

Wound assessment has been discussed in depth above. This section will examine the usual differences between arterial and venous ulcers (see Table 8.4).

It should be noted that ulcers with a rolled edge or raised ulcer base might be malignant.

Referrals

The vast majority of ulcers will not require further assessment. In some instances, however, further advice and assessment may be required. These include:

- a significantly reduced ABPI. Discuss with general practitioner the need for vascular referral
- rapid deterioration of the ulcer
- suspected malignancy
- newly diagnosed diabetes mellitus
- signs of contact dermatitis

- cellulitis (refer to GP or nurse prescriber)
- ulcers that fail to respond to treatment after a three-month period.

Some localities have specialist district nurses or tissue viability nurse nurses who may be able to advise in these instances. Other areas will be dependant on consultant referral.

Nursing management

The aim of management is threefold:

1. To heal the ulcer.
2. To treat the underlying condition.
3. To prevent reccurrence.

Local ulcer treatment

The choice of dressing will depend on assessment of the ulcer (see above). In most instances a simple dressing that is capable of maintaining a moist warm environment conducive to healing should be chosen. Excessive exudate should be absorbed. Dressings should be nonadherent, nontoxic, nonallergenic and nonsensitising.

Ulcers should be cleansed only if necessary. This may not be necessary where there is no old dressing material or any exudate. Legs may be washed with warm tap water containing an emollient if desired. Infection control issues (see Chapter 3) need to be addressed if using a communal bucket in a general practice. The bucket must be lined with plastic (new for each patient) to prevent cross-infection. Patients may appreciate the opportunity to wash their leg if unable to shower or bathe.

Ideally the dressing should be changed once a week unless there is excessive exudate, discomfort or bandage slippage (see Chapter 2, Time management). However, the treatment regime should be determined in conjunction with the patient and there will be instances where more frequent changes are necessary (see patient autonomy, Chapter 1).

Contact sensitivity to treatment may occur at any time. Patients with reactions to unknown sensitisers should be referred to a dermatologist for patch testing. In cases of sensitivity, remove the known or potential allergen, apply a simple non-adherent dressing, and elevate and rest the limb. Liaise with the general practitioner or nurse prescriber to prescribe a steroid ointment, as cream may contain sensitisers. Ointment should be applied sparingly twice daily for 2–4 days. Gradually reduce the amount of steroid used to daily over the following 3–4 days, then replace steroid with white soft paraffin emollient.

Assess the pain level at the wound site. If the dressing is causing pain by adherence, change to a less adherent product.

Compression therapy, exercise and elevation may relieve the pain of patients who have venous ulceration. Analgesia should be tailored to meet individual patient requirements. In extreme cases opiate analgesia may be required.

All patients should be offered accessible and appropriate information on their leg ulcer disease. This should include the rationale for treatment, self-help strategies, services available to them, dietary and lifestyle advice. Many manufacturing companies produce comprehensive patient booklets that can be obtained from representatives. Pharmaceutical company websites offer information on wound care products that can be downloaded for nurse and patient use. Consider using your own educational and health promotion skills (see Chapter 4).

Treating the underlying condition

This is the most important part in leg ulcer treatment. Unless the underlying condition is treated the ulcer is unlikely to respond to treatment.

Venous ulceration

Once arterial involvement has been excluded, the underlying venous disorder should be treated with compression bandaging, exercise and elevation.

Exercise

Walking will exercise the calf muscle and work the muscle pump increasing venous return. Regular flexion and extension exercises are beneficial in working the calf muscle pump for patients with limited mobility. Exercise aids, such as the C'aire Cush, may also be beneficial. These can be bought at some pharmacies.

Elevation

Patients should be encouraged to elevate their legs above hip height when sitting, to facilitate venous return.

Compression

Graduated compression will assist venous return and improve muscle pump function. The suggested level of compression is between 20–40 mmhg at the ankle to 50% of that value at the knee (Kendrick et al. 1994). A compression bandage should be anchored at the base of the toes, exert maximum compression at the ankle and finish at the knee.

Manufacturers' instructions for application should be followed. Bandages that are incorrectly applied are at best uncomfortable and useless and at worst dangerous. Patients with an ABPI of less than 0.8 must not have compression therapy.

Single layer compression, such as Surepress (Convatec) or Tensopress (Smith and Nephew), should be applied to manufacturers' instructions. Padding may be required under the bandaging to protect the leg, particularly over bony prominences. Patients with an ankle circumference of less than 18cm are not suitable for compression bandaging unless sufficient padding is applied to build up the ankle size.

Multi-layer compression systems should provide adequate padding, adequate compression and sustained compression for at least a week. A weekly dressing change is recommended, unless there is strike-through of exudate or patient discomfort. Only accepted systems should be used. These may come in kit form such as Profore, or separately purchased bandages. All patients should have an ankle circumference taken to ensure that the appropriate bandage regime is selected. Manufacturer's instructions for application should be adhered to and the practitioner must be appropriately trained in the application of multi-layer bandaging.

Short stretch bandages such as Comprilan may also be used to achieve compression, and have a lower resting pressure, which some patients find more comfortable and enhance concordance (Krishnamorthy and Melhuish 2000). Most short stretch bandages are made of 100% washable cotton that means they are suitable for patients sensitive to elastic fibres such as rubber, and are also cost effective.

Only nurses who are trained in application of multi-layer compression bandaging should undertake this task, as incorrect bandaging can result in severe tissue damage (Chapter 1, Accountability).

Arterial and mixed aetiology ulceration

Unless advised to the contrary, for example by a vascular surgeon, mixed aetiology ulcers should be treated as arterial. Compression must not be used on ulcers with a substantial arterial component. Any bandages used should offer light retention only.

Mild exercise and ankle exercise should be encouraged, particularly if the patient is immobile. Rest, analgesia and a suitable dressing such as a hydrocolloid or hydrogel may achieve pain control. Patients with arterial disease, particularly those with an ABPI below 0.75, should be considered for a surgical opinion.

Diabetic and rheumatoid ulceration

These ulcers are often difficult to manage. There is usually substantial arterial involvement arising from the peripheral vascular changes associated with these diseases.

Rheumatoid ulceration may show no signs of circulatory disorders and diabetic ulceration may be complicated by peripheral neuropathy. If either of these conditions are suspected but undiagnosed, medical opinion should be sought. Both groups of ulcer should be treated as arterial with rest, pain control, monitoring of the associated disease and early consultant referral.

Preventing recurrence

Advice to prevent ulcer recurrence is essential. Approximately 75% of patients will suffer from recurrence, which can be reduced if appropriate advice is given.

Patients should be advised to report any new damage to legs as soon as possible so treatment can begin. Patients with venous disease require compression therapy for life. When healing is complete they should be measured for suitable hosiery. There are a variety of socks and stockings to meet the needs of most men and women, with made-to-measure hosiery also available. Accurate measurements of ankle, calf and thigh are essential.

Concordance is more likely with below-knee stockings that are relatively easy to put on. Although class 3 stockings (compression 25–35 mmhg) are desirable, a patient with dexterity problems may be encouraged to comply by moving down to class 2 (compression 18–24 mmhg). Patients should be encouraged to continue with exercise and follow a healthy lifestyle. Encourage protection of legs from trauma damage and continue to monitor the underlying disease. New stockings should be prescribed every six months following repeat Doppler testing, to maintain compression that has been lost through washing old hosiery.

Activity 8.2

Undertake an audit of patients with leg ulcers. How many are recurrent? Have they had a Doppler investigation? If the ulcers are venous, has the patient been measured for long-term compression hosiery? If you are unsure about compression hosiery, consider liasing with your community nursing colleagues.

Summary

Individual healing rates will vary whatever the wound or underlying condition. Patients on chemotherapy who present with post-operative wounds can take months to heal. The nurse should discuss an individualised care plan with all patients, including realistic expected healing times and rationale for treatment. Some patients and carers appreciate the opportunity to self-care in conjunction with practice visits. Treatment may need to be changed or the patient may require further investigations or referral to either a consultant or specialist nurse.

As there are constant developments in wound care, the nurse has a responsibility to keep abreast of new evidence through training and liaison with their wound care colleagues.

This chapter provides guidelines to optimise wound healing but experience of working with many wounds, and trying to achieve rapid healing, will be the greatest guide.

Key points

- It is important to keep up to date with new treatment methods but at the same time to acknowledge any limitations in wound management and to refer the patient for specialist advice if necessary.
- The patient's role in the management of their wound should be appreciated and they should be involved in the planning of their care and future management, including self-care.
- All wounds are unique and will respond differently to treatments.

References

Angeras MH, Brandberg A, Falk A & Seeman T (1991) Comparison between sterile saline and tap water for the cleansing of acute traumatic soft tissue wounds. *European Journal of Surgery* 158(33), 347–350.

Barnhorst DA & Barner HB (1968) Prevalence of congenitally absent foot pulses. *New England Journal of Medicine* 278, 264–265.

Biosurgical Research Unit (2003) *LarvE: Method of Application.* www.larve.com/copy

British National Formulary (2007) *BNF 54 September 2007.* Bedfordshire: Pharmaceutical Press.

Cherry GW & Ryan TJ (1985) Enhanced wound angiogenisis with a new hydrocolloid dressing. In TJ Ryan (Ed.) *An Environment for Healing. The Role of Occlusion. International Congress and Symposium. Series no. 88.* London: Royal Society of Medicine.

Chrintz H (1989) Need for surgical wound dressings. *British Journal of Surgery 76*, 204–205.

Cooper R (2004) *A Review of the Evidence for the Use of Topical Antimicrobial Agents in Wound Care.* www.worldwidewounds.com

Cooper R & Lawrence JC (1996) The isolation and identification of bacteria from wounds. *Journal of Wound Care* 5(7), 335–340.

Cutting K (2003) A dedicated follower of fashion? Topical medications and wounds. In R White (Ed.) *The Silver Book.* London: Quay Books.

David J (1986) *Wound Management. A Comprehensive Guide to Dressing and Healing.* London: Martin Dunitz.

Draper J (1985) Making the dressing fit the wound. *Nursing Times* 81(4), 32–35.

Dyson M, Young S & Pendle C (1988) Comparison of the effects of moist and dry conditions on dermal repair. *Journal of Investigative Dermatology* 91(5), 435–449.

Evans H (1997) Treatment of last resort. *Nursing Times* 94 (34), 62–65.

Forrest RD (1982) Development of wound therapy from Dark Ages to the present. *Journal Royal Society Medicine* 75(4), 268–273.

Hutchinson JJ & Lawrence JC (1991) Wound infection under occlusive dressings. *Journal of Hospital Infection* 17, 83–84.

Jones M & Champion A (1998) Natures Way. *Nursing Times* 94(34), 75–78.

Kendrick M, Lucker K, Cullum N & Roe B (1994) *Clinical Information Pack. Number 1. The Management of Leg Ulcers in the Community.* Liverpool: University of Liverpool.

Krishnamorthy L & Melhuish J (2000) Shortstretch bandaging. *Journal of Community Nursing* 14(9) (JCN Online Journal).

Lawrence JC (1997) Wound Irrigation. *Journal of Wound Care* 6(1), 23–26.

Lock PM (1980) The effect of temperature on mitotic activity at the edge of experimental wounds. In A Lundgren & AB Soner (Eds) *Symposia on Wound Healing; Plastic, Surgical and Dermatologic Aspects.* Sweden: Molndal.

Miller M & Dyson M (1996) *The Principles of Wound Care.* London: Macmillan Magazines.

Mimms For Nurses (2006) *District Nurse Formulary.* Southall: Haymarket.

Molan P (2001) *Honey as a Topical Antibacterial Agent for Treatment of Infected Wounds.* www.worldwidewounds.com

Morgan D (1987) *Formulary of Wound Management Products.* Cardiff: Whitchurch Hospital.

Morgan D (1994) *Formulary of Wound Management Products 6th Edn.* Haselmere: Euromed Communications.

Morris C (2006) Wound management and dressing selection. *Wound Essentials* 1, 178–183.

Myers JA (1982) Wound healing and the use of a modern surgical dressing. *The Pharmaceutical Journal* 229(6186), 103–104.

Newman V, Allwood M & Oakes R (1989) The use of metronidazole gel to control the smell of malodorous lesions. *Palliative Medicine* 3(4), 303–305.

Reid J & Morison M (1994) Towards a consensus classification of pressure sores. *Journal of Wound Care* 3(3), 293–294.

Sherman RA (1998) Maggott debridement in Modern Medicine. *Infectious Medicine* 15(9), 651–656.

Silver IA (1985) Oxygen and tissue repair. In TJ Ryan (Ed.) *An Environment for Healing: The Role of Occlusion. International Congress and Symposium. Series No 88.* London: Royal Society of Medicine.

Stewart J (2002) *New Generation Products for Wound Management.* www.worldwidewounds.com

Thomas S (1990) *Wound Management and Dressings.* London: The Pharmaceutical Press.

Thomas S (2004) *MRSA and the Use of Silver Dressings: Overcoming Bacterial Resistance.* www.worldwidewounds.com

Thomas S & Jones M (2005) *Maggots and the battle against MRSA.* Bridgend: Zoobiotic.

Thomas S, Jones M & Andrews A (1998) The use of larval therapy in wound management. *Journal of Wound Care* 7(10), 521–524.

Thomas S, Andrews A, Hay N & Bourgoise S (1999) The antimicrobial activity of maggot secretions: results of a preliminary study. *Journal of Tissue Viability* 9(4), 127–132.

White R (2003) *The Silver Book.* London: Quay Books.

Winter G (1962) Formation of the scab and the rate of epithelialization of superficial wounds in the skin of the young domestic pig. *Nature* 193, 293–294.

Chapter 9

Moving Practice Nursing Forward

Marilyn Edwards

The future for practice nurses who wish to develop and expand their role continues to be dynamic. The changing nature of practice nursing over recent years relates chiefly to the development of health policies. The role has developed from delegated task orientation within a treatment room to professional nursing with specialist skills and knowledge to meet these demands. Universities are constantly revising the education and training requirements of nurses to enable the autonomous practice nurse in 2008 to meet this changing and challenging role. This final chapter examines some of the more recent developments in the changing role of the practice nurse.

Nursing in practice

Practice nurses are generally level one nurses, employed by general practitioners to perform clinical and preventative healthcare procedures in the surgery. According to Rashid, Watts, Lenehan & Haslam (1996), a practice nurse works with a general practitioner (GP) and is responsible for implementing prescribed programmes of care under the supervision of the GP. A modern definition may read 'a practice nurse works with medical and nursing colleagues to devise and implement programmes of healthcare for a defined population'.

Nurses have often been the first point of contact for patients. The number of practice nurses is increasing, with an expected rise in the ratio of nurses to GPs from 60 per 100 to 70 per 100 by 2007 (Cross 2006). Numbers rose from 17,898 in 1196 to 23,797 in 2006 (The Information Centre 2007).

Paniagua (2001) aptly notes that practice nurses continue to develop services and deliver quality care despite political confusion. The enhanced practice nurse role should not be a replacement for medical care, but as a complementary role to the traditional medical model of care. Nurses support doctors in many ways, including the need to improve access to primary care

The Informed Practice Nurse, Edwards, M. (2008), Chichester: Wiley.

(Department of Health 2002). The New General Medical Services (GMS) Contract lays a greater emphasis on health prevention and health promotion than previous contracts (National Health Service Confederation/BMA 2003); this role is primarily the remit of the nursing team.

Practice nurses are often autonomous, innovative and self-motivated, moving from novice to expert, but for some nurses the role is a job and not a career. This will be reflected in the motivation to study, especially if self-funding is required. However, there is a need for purely clinical nurses within the workforce. *Agenda for Change* (Department of Health 2004) may be an incentive for career development, as it recognises individual knowledge and skills, although some GPs may be slower than others to embrace this concept until it is mandatory.

Nurse-led management in clinical care

Where there is a team of nurses, each may have a specialist interest; this does not however, make them a specialist nurse. They can, however, be a valuable resource to both nursing and medical colleagues.

The current health policy involves the increasing transfer of healthcare services from secondary to primary care. This builds on the continuing increase in practice nurse workload over the past decade. Most patients with diabetes, respiratory disease and coronary heart disease are managed in primary care, with only difficult patients referred to secondary care, although the level of primary care varies between and within practices and localities.

Nurses who have a special interest in a condition can develop the expertise to provide further services within primary care, for example sexual health, dermatology and minor surgery. They may also be involved in ENT, orthopaedics, urology and gynaecology, if the practice decides to offer these services (see practice based commissioning later in chapter). The challenge will be in juggling the expanding workload within the allocated hours. It is questionable whether there are sufficient experienced nurses to deliver a range of enhanced services as well as the *Quality Outcomes and Frameworks* requirements (British Medical Association 2004), hence the value of skill mix.

Skill mix

The term grade mix is thought more appropriate than skill mix to describe a team where members have mixed skills and expertise (Smith 1993). For convenience, this text will refer to skill mix. Skill can be defined in terms of a number of variables such as experience, knowledge or qualifications (Richardson & Maynard 1995).

Skill mix can be applied throughout general practice, as the continuing shift from secondary to primary care has led to a corresponding increase in community nurse and medical workload. This includes pre-operative assessments, and managing post-operative wound infections. GPs rely on skill mix to deliver quality primary care, especially in areas where GPs are difficult to recruit, and nurses are expected to fill the gap. Nursing roles in general practice must develop to meet the needs of the practice within an increasingly limited budget.

Healthcare assistants

As the practice nurse role has expanded to encompass more of the chronic disease management, triage and prescribing, there has been a drive to employ more healthcare assistants (HCAs) to support the nursing team. This appears to be a logical decision, as appropriately trained HCAs can share the workload. Many HCAs come into general practice from secondary care, phlebotomy and from working as a general practice receptionist. Their experience will vary greatly, but a thorough induction course and support from their practice nurse mentor should ensure safe practice.

Facilities in localities will vary, but NVQ training packages are available, and HCA staff should be encouraged and supported to access this training. The current NHS funding crisis may restrict training opportunities for all staff, resulting in the need for in-house training. It is recognised that practice staff will need support to take on these supportive roles (Cross 2006). This is an ideal opportunity for practice nurses to update their knowledge and utilise their teaching skills. Scottish practice nurses identified opportunities and threats in developing the role of the HCA (Burns 2006). Opportunities included the provision of cost-effective care, developing teamwork and the chance to nurture the HCA career prospects, while threats included role boundaries, clarity of line management and the fear of time together with nurse and HCA not being protected.

Box 9.1 lists some of the tasks that can be delegated to the HCA following adequate training. HCAs should work within defined protocols and not be placed in a position where they are required to make clinical judgements (Royal College of Nursing 2007a). The HCA is directly accountable to a registered healthcare professional and should have regular supervision and assessment of competence. The registered nurse, in turn, is accountable for the appropriate delegation of any task. The *Working In Partnership Programme* (Wipp) enables both the HCA and qualified nurse to examine and develop

---

Box 9.1   Tasks that can be delegated to the HCA include:

- phlebotomy
- sterilising instruments (although many are now disposable)
- simple dressings
- routine blood pressure recordings
- weighing patients
- urinalysis
- stock control and ordering
- chaperoning
- new patient health checks
- 24-hour blood pressure recordings
- ECGs
- smoking cessation
- spirometry
- assisting in minor surgery
- ear irrigation.

---

their own competencies (Hopkins, Hughes & Vaughan 2007). See Useful addresses at the end of the chapter for the contact details.

An appropriately trained HCA should understand the implications of abnormal weight, blood pressure and urinalysis readings, and be able to identify a wound that is deteriorating and report this to nursing colleagues for action. The RCN (2007a) noted that HCAs are used inappropriately within general practice. One anecdotal example of this is HCAs who are expected by the GP to undertake contraceptive pill checks prior to generating a prescription. This raises many concerns about safe practice, as this consultation should involve more than a mere blood pressure reading. As well as assessing concordance with medication and addressing any specific concerns the woman may have, this is also an opportunity for a discussion on sexual health, cervical smears or preconception advice (see Chapter 4, Health promotion).

Wiltshire FHSA introduced a clinical nurse assistant (CNA) post as a trial in one fund-holding general practice in 1993 (Fairfield 1996). Following NVQ level 3 training the CNA was able to undertake treatment room tasks previously undertaken by a G grade nurse or reception staff. The practice subsequently reduced the number of G grade hours. This scenario could suggest that the G grade nurse was over-skilled for that role (see Chapter 2, Management).

The benefits of employing an HCA in general practice will depend on each nurse's perception. It could be argued that registered nurses are doing themselves a disservice by encouraging skill mix. Will the HCA role devalue the practice nurse role, or will it enable the practice nurse to use their skills more effectively? There is no doubt that many practice nurses are over-qualified for some tasks they have traditionally undertaken. Less skilled nurses should be used to assist, not replace, qualified nurses. This is particularly relevant as doctors devolve much of their chronic disease management to practice nurses. However, it must be recognised that clinical judgement is a vital component of all nursing interventions, from urinalysis and weight checks to hypertension monitoring. HCAs will not have the assessment skills or experience that nurses have attained through years of practice. If they are expected to undertake these tasks should they therefore consider nurse training?

Cooper (1997) described how the introduction of a clinical assistant within her general practice led to a flexible practice team. The assistant received on-going training that allowed her to develop skills from clerical support to clinical tasks. Practices may already have unofficial healthcare assistants by virtue of their reception/clerical staff undertaking many of the tasks for which Cooper's assistant was employed. A trained HCA can complement the practice nurse to offer a cost-effective service to patients, enhancing the job satisfaction of both roles. The RCN views skill mix as a more appropriate use of nursing skills than merely a cost-cutting exercise (RCN 1997a). RCN guidelines for HCAs are listed in Box 9.2.

Box 9.2   Recommendations for healthcare assistants (HCAs) (RCN 1997a):

- HCAs should have been trained to NVQ level 3
- patients must be aware of differences between a nurse and an HCA
- delegated tasks should be appropriate and take account of individual abilities
- procedures needing nursing skills and clinical judgement should not be delegated to an HCA
- results of clinical measurements should be reported to a nurse or doctor for a decision on a course of action
- a system will be in place to ensure that concerns about practice standards can be reported and action taken.

Treatment room nurses

Registered nurses might choose to work purely as treatment room nurses and undertake all the clinical tasks in Box 9.1. They might have some involvement in chronic disease management, supporting the lead nurse. They also have the advantage of being able to administer injections, undertake cervical cytology, assess wounds and support HCAs within their role. Although some nurses may wish to remain in this role, others will take an interest in a specific disease area and begin the voyage of study and development. It is understandable that some nurses may feel threatened and anxious by skill mix, as lower grades appear to be a more economic option for employers who are looking for creative skill and grade mix, as they are no longer reimbursed for staff wages. It may, however, be in the practice's interest to employ more, rather than less, experienced nurses to cope with the shortage of doctors, and to meet the *Quality Outcomes and Frameworks* requirements (British Medical Association 2004).

Specialist practitioner

The United Kingdom Central Council (UKCC) recognised that general practice nursing encompasses a wide range of nursing skills, and was an area that required a specialist qualification (UKCC 1994a). The Registrar's letter (UKCC 1994b) laid out the standards required for post-registration education leading to the qualification of specialist practitioner. This enabled practitioners to exercise higher levels of judgement and discretion in clinical care (Box 9.3). Patients and clients should have access to specialist care wherever nursing care is given, although not all practitioners need become specialists.

Box 9.3   Standards required for specialist practice

Specialist practitioners are expected to:

- demonstrate higher levels of clinical decision making
- monitor and improve standards of care through supervision of practice
- undertake clinical audit
- provide skilled professional leadership
- develop practice through research
- teach and support professional colleagues.

The UKCC and National Boards published a statement in June 1996 that aimed to clarify the position in respect to the use of the title *specialist practitioner* (UKCC 1996). A specialist qualification, which is recorded on the Nursing and Midwifery Council (NMC) register, can be obtained by undertaking a first degree programme at a higher education institute. Institutions approved for these programmes have Assessment of Prior Learning mechanisms in place to ensure maximum credit is offered for appropriate prior learning and learning from experience (APEL). This course can include a module for nonmedical prescribing that allows the nurse to prescribe from a limited formulary (see later).

Nurse practitioner

Currently any nurse is free to use the title of nurse practitioner, although the UKCC stated in the final report on PREP that it did not recognise the term nurse practitioner, as all nurses are practitioners in their own right (UKCC 1993).

Castledine (1995) defined a nurse practitioner as: 'A registered nurse who has been specially prepared to carry out and integrate a more medical model of care into his/her nursing practice, with the purpose of improving health assessment, management and delivery of services at the first level of access.'

Development of the nurse practitioner

The nurse practitioner (NP) was introduced in the United States of America during the late 1960s in response to a shortage of physicians, and was very much a doctor substitute role. Barbara Stilwell pioneered the role in the United Kingdom in the 1970s, in the firm belief that the NP would advance the contribution of nursing within primary healthcare. The NP was initially involved in five key areas of work (see Box 9.4).

Box 9.4   The five key areas of work of the nurse practitioner (Stilwell 1984)

The nurse practitioner:

1. acts as an alternative consultant for the patient
2. detects serious disease by physical examination
3. manages minor and chronic ailments and injuries
4. provides health education
5. counsels.

The role of the NP in the UK developed from government concerns about cost effectiveness in healthcare highlighted by the *Neighbourhood Nursing, a Focus for Care* report (Department of Health 1986). Studies by Stilwell, Greenfield, Drury and Hull (1987) and Stilwell (1988) concluded that when given a choice between a NP and a medical practitioner, most patients chose a consultation with the NP appropriately and the NP provided care that is equivalent to, and sometimes more effective, than physicians, particularly in the care of patients with chronic disease. NPs are not a cheap alternative to physicians, as although cheaper to employ their consultations are usually longer.

The role of the NP has been recognised as being a means towards improving primary healthcare, particularly with relation to client choice, satisfaction and the inequalities that exist in service provision and usage (Whitehead 1988). Nurse practitioners have been instrumental in reducing some of the inequalities in health both in less developed countries and among disadvantaged groups in the UK, demonstrated by the frequent reports in nursing journals about healthcare for the homeless.

The role of NP may vary between practitioners, but is likely to have expanded to encompass a caring rather than a medical curing role. Many practice nurses will be undertaking this role although may not be calling themselves NPs. The practice nurse working as a NP could offer patients an alternative to a GP consultation, although it may be argued that the role falls within a medical remit. GPs vary in their acceptance of nurses in this role; innovative GPs actively encourage nurse practitioner education, while others will feel threatened.

Marsh and Dawes (1995) demonstrated that appropriately trained nurses are competent to diagnose and manage minor illnesses in general practice. Half of the patients in their study only required advice on self-care, with or without recommendation for over-the-counter drugs. NPs can improve the quality and choice within primary care by offering patients a choice of professional and consultation style (Fawcett Henesy & West 1995). It is probable that many experienced practice nurses are currently undertaking this role unofficially. There is a clear role for both doctors and nurses, with complementary skills, when roles and responsibilities are clearly defined.

The RCN clarified some of the issues surrounding the title and role of the nurse practitioner, believing that only those nurses who have completed a course of specific education for the role should use the title (RCN 1997b). The criteria for identifying a nurse practitioner are listed in Box 9.5, demonstrating an expansion of the role from Box 9.4.

One study examined several randomised controlled trials comparing doctor/nurse substitution (RCN 2004). Although nurse consultations were longer, patients received more information about their health and illness

---

Box 9.5   The trained nurse practitioner (RCN 1997b)

The trained nurse practitioner:

- manages his/her own caseload
- has undertaken a specific course of study to at least first degree level
- makes professionally autonomous decisions
- assesses the healthcare needs of previously undiagnosed patients
- screens patients/clients for disease risk factors and early signs of disease
- negotiates a healthcare plan with the patient/client
- counsels and offers health education
- refers to other healthcare providers.

---

from nurses than doctors. Prescribing costs were similar. Requests for clinical investigations varied between studies. The overall results highlighted increased patient satisfaction of care in their consultation and management by nurses/nurse practitioners. These results are supported by Seale (2006), who compared NP and GP consultations. NPs are also reported to be valued for their listening and explanation skills (Macdonald 2005).

Not all GPs are comfortable with the advanced role of the NP. There is a fear that the doctor–patient relationship will diminish and the NP role will undermine general practice as a profession (Alcolado 2000). The expertise of the primary care NP is parallel to that of a GP, operating as a *specialist generalist* (RCN 1997b). NPs offer an alternative source of care that is complementary to the GP. They should not be treated as doctor substitutes.

Advanced nurse practitioners

Advanced nursing practice was stated to be:

... concerned with adjusting the boundaries for the development of future practice, pioneering and developing new roles responsive to changing needs and with advancing clinical practice, research and education to enrich professional practice as a whole. (UKCC 1994a)

However, this definition is controversial, as advanced nursing practice is an umbrella term for a range of emerging nursing roles (Wilson & Bunnell 2007).

Advanced Nurse Practitioners (ANPs) have developed to meet the complex demands of current healthcare systems. The ANP course is at Masters level, and has then the option of a nonmedical prescribing module that qualifies the nurse to prescribe from the whole British National Formulary (see later).

The NMC (2005) consultation document on regulating advanced level registration suggested ANPs had four key responsibilities:

- taking responsibility for case management
- making differential diagnosis
- planning and providing care and treatment, including prescribing medication, in collaboration with others, as appropriate
- providing health education, counselling and leadership

This appears similar to NP criteria, but including more advanced assessment and diagnostic skills. A study by Carnwell and Daly (2003) revealed the practice nurse ANPs' expertise lay in their advanced practical assessment and diagnosis of patients, but they had little opportunity for strategic development. Although practice nurse ANPs needed longer appointment times than doctors, they reduced pressure on GPs by freeing up their time to deal with more complex problems, reducing waiting times, being an appropriate gender (primarily for women's health) and reducing the need for a locum. Use of ANPs for 'mundane' work was, however, seen to restrict future development of their role. It was noted that having an ANP in practice could raise patients' expectations of the role of other nurses. Good communication should prevent this occurring. ANPs described their direct-patient care role as more holistic, emphasising patient education in self-care.

Unfortunately, participants in this study were often paid at the same grade as a practice nurse, which could be viewed as a major deterrent to a nurse considering undertaking a Masters course.

Gaining an ANP qualification should not automatically detract from the other nursing skills that might enhance a consultation. Patients benefit from the unique skills offered by advanced nurses and those with specialist qualifications, as they receive both nursing and a degree of medical intervention simultaneously (Wilson & Bunnell 2007).

Lorentzon and Hooker (2006) stressed that what a person fulfilling the various roles is called is unimportant, as long there is a common understanding within the primary care team and among patients about the skills and functions of the individual. This can be achieved through publicity within the practice newsletter, practice website and/or a photoboard located in the reception area.

Table 9.1   A hypothetical grade mix which reflects skill or expertise

Role	Grade
Advanced nurse practitioner/nurse practitioner	H/I (AfC 7/8) team leader, prescriber
2 Practice nurses	F/G grade (AfC 6) skilled practitioners with special interest in at least one chronic disease area
Practice nurse	E grade (AfC 5) treatment room nurse
HCA	B/C grade (AfC 3/4) trained to meet practice needs and assist other grades
(AfC = Agenda for Change)	

Table 9.1 offers a hypothetical skill and grade mix, which reflects the expertise of the practitioner. This would not be feasible where only one or two nurses are employed. Combinations of expertise should reflect the needs of the practice.

Activity 9.1

Undertake a strengths, weaknesses, opportunities and threats (SWOT) analysis of skill mix (grade mix) in your workplace. Discuss this with your team and gain agreement to overcome the weaknesses and threats. An example of a SWOT analysis is shown in Figure 9.1.

Nonmedical prescribing (nurse prescribing)

The concept of nurse prescribing evolved from *Neighbourhood Nursing, a Focus for Care* (Department of Health 1986), which initially allowed nurses with a district nurse and health visiting qualification to prescribe from a very limited formulary. The *Crown Report* (Department of Health 1989) defined three areas in which nurses would be able to prescribe (Box 9.6).

Many nurses prescribe unofficially, for example in managing chronic disease and wound care, although this is illegal practice. The nurse prescribing qualification was seen to formalise proxy prescribing for the nurses in one cohort in 2003–2004 (Bradley, Campbell & Nolan 2005), which may be an incentive for nurses to undertake the course.

All community nurses are now eligible to access a prescribing course, providing they have first level registration, have been qualified for more than three years, and can study at level 3. The course can be either the V100 as

Strengths	Weaknesses
HCA can undertake routine blood pressure readings	HCA may not understand implication of reading
Cost-effective patient care	Need time to train new staff
Opportunities	**Threats**
Employ a treatment room nurse	May be used by employer to downgrade nursing staff salaries
Train new staff to undertake specific role, e.g. smoking cessation	

Figure 9.1 An example of a SWOT analysis.

Box 9.6   Areas in which nurses would be able to prescribe (Department of Health 1989)

- Initial prescribing from a limited list of items – the Nurses' Formulary
- Supplying medicines within group protocols, e.g. immunisations
- Adjust timing and dosage of medication prescribed by a medical practitioner within clearly defined protocols.

---

part of the specialist practitioner qualification, or as a stand-alone module, V300 Independent and Supplementary prescribing. The V100 does not attract any academic credits but allows the nurse to prescribe from the nurse formulary. This is of limited value in the management of most chronic diseases. The V300 usually attracts 30 credits at level 3, and allows the nurse wider

---

Box 9.7 Benefits of nurse prescribing

For the nurse:

- a service which is more appropriate and responsive to patient needs
- better, faster, more cost-effective treatment of minor but potentially serious and therefore costly conditions
- more appropriate use of nurses' extensive professional skills
- increased nurse autonomy and satisfaction
- increased awareness of prescribing costs
- increased awareness of over-the-counter (OTC) products
- saving on GP appointment time
- improved working relationship with medical colleagues.

For the patient:

- saving patient time
- providing a complete package of care
- provision of more responsive patient care
- better medicine management increases patient safety.

---

prescribing power. Some of the advantages of nurse prescribing for the nurse and the patient are listed in Box 9.7.

When prescribing, supplying or altering the timing or dosage of an item, nurses have the opportunity to actively engage in health teaching and question whether any prescription is required at all. Nurses have the communication skills to discuss risk/benefits of treatment and assess concordance. Although many more medications are becoming available over the counter, members of the public expect infinitely more knowledge and expertise from a nurse who prescribes than when choosing a product for themselves.

The *NHS Plan* (Department of Health 2000) stated that the majority of nurses should be able to prescribe from an extended formulary. Nurse prescribing sends a powerful message to the public and others that nursing is not subservient to medicine (Reid 2003). Practice nurses may be unwilling to undertake this training for several reasons, including the lack of financial reward for the increased responsibility, even though they recognise the benefits to the patients. It could be argued that nurse prescribing is essential to complement chronic disease management in offering a holistic care package for patients. As noted above, many nurses write prescriptions for the doctor to sign, especially in wound care management. In this instance, the signing doctor takes responsibility for the prescription.

Since 1 May 2006, Independent and Supplementary prescribers can prescribe all licensed medications in the British National Formulary, for any medication within their clinical competence, with the exception of some controlled drugs (Department of Health 2006a). For example, a respiratory nurse would not usually prescribe for a mental health problem. It is expected that controlled drugs will be included in the criteria in the near future.

Bradley et al.'s cohort (2005) was concerned that they would not receive the support they needed following qualification; nurses have a responsibility to continue their development. Standards of proficiency for nurse prescribers have been set by the NMC, and include the requirement for continued professional development (NMC 2006). Attending GP/nurse prescribing meetings, accessing prescribing websites, or asking the PCT pharmacist for support could fulfill this requirement.

It has been suggested that experienced nurse prescribers could mentor students as an alternative to doctors, as one way to address the shortage of medical mentors (Learner 2006). This may be feasible in the future, when practice nurses are experienced, but realistically it is more likely that current practice nurse prescribers will require support from their GPs.

Readers who are interested in undertaking nurse prescribing are recommended to contact their local university for course information, and access relevant websites listed at the end of this chapter.

Patient Group Directions (PGDs)

Group protocols were widely used as an arrangement by which nurses could administer vaccinations in general practice without a doctor writing an individual prescription. However, these were often unclear and deemed illegal, with a potential risk of prosecution for anyone supplying or administering prescription-only medicines (POM) using this system (RCN 2007b). Group protocols were replaced with PGDs following legislative changes in 2000.

PGDs relate to the supply and administration of a POM to a person or group of people (RCN 2007b). A written direction is usually prepared and signed by a PCT pharmacist and doctor, by the employing GP and each nurse who will give the medicine. Commonly used PGDs include those for childhood immunisations, travel and influenza vaccinations. The nurse assesses the patient's need without necessarily referring back to a doctor for an individual prescription. PGDs should be updated regularly, and are a legal requirement for practice. This can cause difficulties when a new vaccine is launched, and no PGD has been prepared. In this instance individual prescriptions should be obtained. Nurses are encouraged to keep a folder of updated PGDs to hand, and use them as reference. This can be very useful for reference when fielding patient/parents queries about side effects of new or unfamiliar vaccines.

Triage

A definition of triage is:

sorting out; allocation of resources to where they will have the most effect, rather than to where the need is most urgent or severe. (Chambers 2006)

Appropriately trained nurses are competent to diagnose and manage minor illnesses, and undertake triage in general practice (White 2001). This role has evolved over time, and experienced nurses are undertaking these roles without formal training, although they usually have the necessary competencies. Nurses have the expertise and autonomy for this role, which supports the doctors and offers patients an enhanced service.

An appropriately triaged patient may be referred to the HCA for routine blood pressure measurement, the practice nurse for chronic disease management, the NP/ANP for minor illness or differential diagnosis, and the GP for other conditions.

Nurse triage has been shown to be as safe as general practitioner delivered alternatives, and is reported to reduce same-day GP activity by between 25% and 49% (Richards et al. 2004). Benefits of triage include diverting appointments from same day to routine, thus allowing staff to plan their workload, and patients having their concerns discussed with a healthcare professional in minutes rather than days. Disadvantages include busier same-day surgeries and increased nursing time.

Most nurses will have been asked by reception staff to answer patients' queries about whether or not they need to see a doctor. Examples of triage may include answering telephone calls relating to the management of influenza or diarrhoea, a family planning trained nurse offering advice on missed contraceptive pills, or managing walk-in minor injuries. The ever-increasing workload of doctors and nurses has made nurse triage an important part of service provision.

A recent study by Connechen and Walter (2006) concluded that telephone triage is an appropriate method of dealing with requests for same-day appointments, resulting in high patient satisfaction. They assert that successful telephone triage is dependent on nurses having specialised training and good judgement. However, Richards et al. (2004) suggest that many nurses are trained in-house by GPs, and do not have specialist practitioner qualifications. An audit of telephone consultations can be used to review practice and support clinical supervision (Richards et al. 2004) (see Chapter 2, Management). Experienced nurses may find specialised training helpful in formalising their activities, although, as discussed above, funding and training may be difficult to access.

One study investigated practice nurse management of minor illness (Shum et al. 2000). The participant nurses were trained to degree level on an accredited course and supported by their GPs.

Although nurse consultations were slightly longer than those by a GP, nurses offered more advice on self-medication and general self-management. There was a high level of patient satisfaction following nurse consultations and the authors concluded that the practice nurse seemed to offer an effective service for patients with minor illness who requested a same-day appointment.

Minor illness management training, supported by computerised management protocols, will enhance nurse triage in general practice.

The primary healthcare team

The primary healthcare team (PHCT) (see Figure 9.2) has now expanded to include community matrons and intermediate care team members. This wider team offers the opportunity for improved communication and an understanding of each person's role. Although it is difficult to get all team members together for a quarterly meeting, the benefits of these meetings are enormous. Putting faces to names and exchanging information about patients and services is invaluable. It is worthwhile asking team members who cannot attend for feedback on current activities, innovative practice, or areas of concern that the practice could address. Sending copies of the minutes to each member to keep them abreast of any new practice developments is also recommended.

Training

Primary Care Trusts and/or employers should provide study days for mandatory updates, but these do not necessarily meet the training needs of individual nurses. Although there is a practice staff training budget, this is restricted and may cover only mandatory training for nurses, such as child protection, immunisation updates and cervical cytology training and updates. Problems can arise when a lack of flexibility may prevent more than one nurse from a practice attending an update, particularly when no alternative dates or venues are available. It is reasonable to expect nurses to share

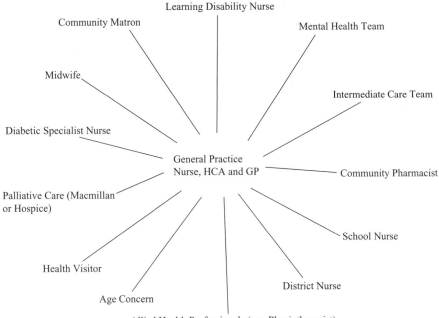

Figure 9.2 An example of a Primary Healthcare Team.

knowledge with their colleagues when this occurs. Study days commissioned through private companies are often expensive but are usually more flexible.

PREP has made it compulsory for nurses to constantly advance their practice through learning, but certificated learning experience is not required. Reading and reflection are included within Professional education and Practice (PREP). Multi-professional in-house training is valuable when topics include specific areas of disease processes and patient management, especially when discussing practice protocols and NICE guidelines. This can be particularly helpful when trying to devise protocols for complex conditions such as chronic kidney disease, when patients will require both medical and nursing support. It is incumbent on nurses to request training and suggest multi-disciplinary training with their medical colleagues.

A variety of courses are now available through academic centres and via open learning. E-learning, via the internet, increases study opportunities if nurses are sufficiently motivated to use this method. These include academic degrees, diplomas and certificates for chronic diseases and areas of special interest. Nurses should ensure that study leave is incorporated into their contract of employment, as it is for general practitioners.

Nurses must seize every opportunity to ensure they are appropriately trained to meet their expanding roles. This can be achieved by:

1. identifying your training needs at your annual appraisal and negotiating study leave
2. contacting Higher Education institutes for a prospectus of relevant courses
3. negotiating funding with the practice manager – this may require some commitment from yourself
4. if in doubt, liase with the practice nurse facilitator/trainer at the PCT.

Agenda for Change is viewed as a key element in ensuring all staff have a career structure, with support for the process of appraisal and development of staff (RCN 2005). With an ageing practice nurse population, there is a clear need to recruit and retain staff through good employment practice which includes training opportunities.

Reflective practice

Critical reflection has been described as a positive journey of self-discovery (Ashby 2006). Although some nurses may view reflective practice negatively, it can be cathartic, especially for those who work in isolation. Many nurses focus on continued action but devote little time to reflect on this action. Reflection is essential if innovation in nursing practice is to replace traditional methods of care. The issues raised throughout this book are intended to encourage the reader to reflect on their current practice using simple and useful learning exercises. All outcomes should be viewed as a positive learning experience.

Reflection is an integral part of development, and includes reflecting on any study undertaken. Attending a study day does not provide evidence of professional development; the nurse must reflect whether the session met their aims, what they have learned, and how their practice will change. It may simply be that the session reinforced their current knowledge, which may enhance job satisfaction. On other occasions, it can be an impetus to change practice or rewrite practice policies and protocols to effect change (see Chapter 2).

Reflection is also invaluable within clinical supervision or during peer discussion, where scenarios can be discussed and evaluated. Reflection also includes good practice, which is worth sharing with colleagues.

Nurses who were critically reflective were reported to be sufficiently confident and empowered to question their own practice and that of others

(Ashby 2006). The unreflective practitioner is deemed potentially dangerous as they may not recognise and therefore learn by their mistakes.

Activity 9.2

For one week keep a note of any areas of patient care, or interpersonal interaction, on which you can reflect. What was particularly good, and what could have been done better? What were your feelings? Devise an action plan following each reflection. All the experiences should have a positive outcome.

Clinical supervision

Clinical supervision is an interactive process between providers of healthcare that enables the development of professional knowledge and skills (Butterworth and Faugier 1993, cited by National Health Service Executive 1996), with the aim of encouraging professional development and support for nursing staff to ensure a high standard of clinical and managerial practice.

Clinical supervision for practice nurses has not developed in the same way as other nursing disciplines, partly due to the poorly defined role of practice nurses who have no requirement to demonstrate their competence formally. Although some GPs undertake an educative aspect of supervision, delivered through on-the-job training, supportive supervision is rare.

The need for clinical supervision for practice nurses was recognised and addressed in North Staffordshire, where the value of supervision by an experienced practice nurse was demonstrated through a consensus workshop (Cook & Leech 1996). The concept of a group of nurses meeting with a supervisor on a regular monthly basis to discuss a range of topics and offer peer group support could be incorporated into practice nurse groups, especially where nurses work in isolation. In the author's locality, clinical supervision ceased to continue after a couple of sessions due to lack of support from the nurses. This may be because some nurses failed to recognise the benefits of this support, while others were not allowed protected time to attend.

As noted above, reflection on past experiences through discussion offers nurses the opportunity to increase their self-awareness and meet individual professional needs, leading in turn to a higher level of patient care. Clinical supervision offers the opportunity for nurses to critically self-evaluate all aspects of their clinical experiences, including successes and errors.

Nurses may be more comfortable using the term clinical support in place of clinical supervision. Support more accurately describes the concept, while supervision conjures up observation and assessment. It is as important to negotiate time for clinical supervision and reflection as it is for training.

Practice based commissioning

Practice based commissioning (PBC) is a key part of the NHS reforms, offering general practitioners and their nursing colleagues the opportunity to deliver services to meet local patient needs (Department of Health 2006b). Each general practice, or group of practices (local consortia) will mutually agree a PBC plan with their Primary Care Trust. The scheme should allow freedom and flexibility to respond to the population needs, commissioning services for their patients and keeping any profits for reinvestment, although this must be used for 'national or local priorities' (O'Dowd 2006). Nurses were expected to be involved in designing the services, adding their knowledge and skills to the planning process. Although expected to deliver services, nurses' input in commissioning has been conspicuous in its absence, either due to lack of invitation to PBC meetings, or lack of interest from individuals. Although not involved in the planning, there is no doubt that nurses will be heavily involved in the implementation of care delivery.

Nurse partnerships

Nurses and doctors often have conflicting views of partnership, which may relate to the doctor's previous dominant role over the nurse-handmaiden. Partnerships can differ, from total equality, profit sharing only, or part-partnerships. There has been increasing interest in equal partnerships since 1993, when the topic was debated in the 'Heathrow debate' (Department of Health 1993).

Radical changes in primary healthcare were addressed by the Department of Health (1996) in *Choice and Opportunity: Primary Care: the Future*. The traditional structure of GP partnerships was challenged by a suggestion of practice-based contracts that would embrace nonmedical professionals, including nurses. Parkinson (1996) has noted the success of nurse/GP partners.

Nurses can enter into partnerships with GPs, rather than be employed by them (Royal College of Nursing 2005). A nurse partner is in a strong position to manage and influence the development of the general practice and take a more strategic role in healthcare policy. Some personal and professional benefits of being a nurse partner include a sense of ownership and stronger teamwork between nurse partner and GPs, having an equal say in decision making, and financial reward through profit sharing. However, negative aspects of partnership include increased responsibility and financial liability. The need to obtain independent professional legal advice and indemnity is crucial, to protect the nurse in this challenging position.

Ideally GP/community nurse partnerships should be the future of general practice teams. In reality, workload (both paid employment and home/child care) and lack of finance to contribute to a partnership may inhibit many interested nurses from pursuing this course of action.

The future

The future for practice nurses continues to be challenging. GP emergency services have developed throughout the UK to meet the need for out-of-hours medical care. The development and expansion of telephone help line and triage services are expected to reduce surgery visits and GP call-outs, and increase home management of minor illness. However, there is still a group of patients who contact NHS Direct for advice, and then ask to see a doctor or nurse to reinforce the advice.

Private companies running general practices and employing practice nurses may move the emphasis from care to profit, which is an alien concept to most nurses. Currently most practices are small businesses that, although they aim to make a profit, are generally patient orientated.

The Nurse Practitioner and Advanced Nurse Practitioner have the skills working in triage to identify those patients who need to see a nurse or doctor, or who can self-manage at home. Bowles (1995) suggested that nurse practitioners could set up independent practice as primary practitioners, consulting GPs as necessary. This is not an uncommon occurrence, where the nurses with extended roles and responsibilities employ the doctors.

Improved communication and liaison with the wider primary healthcare team can save duplication of services, resulting in an improved patient experience and should be nurtured. The emphasis must be on teamwork and not rivalry within the primary care arena. The role of each professional must be developed to meet the needs of the practice population. Teamwork should improve communication, prevent overlap of services and lead to an improvement of patient care.

Traditionally, the general practitioner largely determined the service the practice nurse offered to the practice population. This has changed. Some of the main changes in doctor/nurse/patient relationships are shown in Box 9.8. Nurses have a wide range of specialised skills and can offer a

---

Box 9.8   Changes in nurse/doctor/patient relationships

Past	2008
nurse was delegated tasks by GP	nurse directs patient care
doctor instructed nurse	doctor asks nurse's advice
doctor taught nurse	nurse trains doctor
nurse was handmaiden to doctor	nurse is a professional equal
for the patient	*for the patient*
patient expects to see doctor	patient chooses to see the nurse
doctor dictated care plan	negotiated/shared management
patient asked doctor/nurse	patient attends with internet data

---

proactive approach to health. They are now in a position to advise the GP on many aspects of patient care, and are often asked about respiratory and diabetic management.

Nurses must constantly be prepared to move into areas of practice that will maximise their skills, and undertake research and evaluation to achieve the best possible health outcome for patients. It is continually stressed that nurses should apply only evidence-based care. However, there is little published research by practice nurses, suggesting that the evidence base used may not always be appropriate to general practice. Research and audits should be shared, and not left on office shelves.

The reader is urged to reflect on an area of practice that interests them, and which may merit research. Anyone planning a research project can contact their PCT research and development committee for guidance; their approval must be sought prior to a study. It is probably more helpful to undertake a research skills module through higher education.

Funding is available from several sources, including scholarships, which are advertised regularly in the nursing press; from an employer, if keen enough about the project; or through pharmaceutical funding. For example, a company selling medication for respiratory diseases, cardiovascular disease or diabetes, might be willing to fund a research project in that area of healthcare. Pharmaceutical representatives will be able to advise on the amount of available funding, if any. Research projects do not have to be major works; it is the relevance to patient care that is important.

The future practice nurse will be a highly trained, autonomous non-medical prescriber, who will offer patients a one-stop shop for holistic care. Triage, both telephone and face-to-face, will be the norm. Nurses will run an increased number of specialist clinics, reducing secondary care referrals and follow-up appointments.

There is an opportunity to expand the traditional role, as demonstrated by practice nurses performing minor surgery (Elton & Bevan 2005). Nurses will be more closely involved in training medical students and registrar doctors in infection control (see Chapter 3), chronic disease management, family planning and women's health. Nurses will become partners in the practice, thus ensuring a greater appreciation of the nurse's role, while the more entrepreneurial nurses will employ doctors.

Summary

Practice nurses make a valuable and major contribution to primary care; therefore professional development and career satisfaction is essential. Higher education to gain a recognised qualification, such as specialist practitioner or advanced nurse practitioner, will increase job satisfaction through greater understanding of the role and opportunities for involvement in strategic planning. However, changes in Primary Care Trust configurations have reduced, and will continue to reduce, the opportunity for nurses to become a nursing voice on professional executive committees. Nurses must be encouraged to develop their role and autonomy within the primary healthcare team and to play a greater part in decision making.

Patients and clients must not be misled, either inadvertently or intentionally; the role of the caregiver should be made clear to a recipient of care, whatever title a practitioner holds or chooses to use.

Resources for the NHS will always be finite, and it is essential to maximise the benefits for patients with the available resources. The primary healthcare team must adapt service provision to meet identified health needs and work together with shared philosophies and objectives.

Practice nurses offer a complementary role, not a replacement, to the traditional medical model of care. Nurses who prefer to practice traditional clinical care skills rather than undertake courses in higher education must not be devalued; high-quality individualised patient care is the mainstay of practice nursing. Nurses must practice at the level for which they are competent and confident. Grade/skill mixes meet this need.

Higher education equips practice nurses to undertake research and clinical audit and offer evidence-based nursing care. Many nurses undertake valuable research and audit projects but do not publish their findings. The reader is encouraged to share knowledge and improve practice. Nurses will then have the evidence with which to face any opposition by an employer when attempting to change practice. In a climate of increasing numbers of litigation actions, nurses must be sufficiently assertive to protect both their patients and their own professional status.

The prospect of GP/nurse partnerships should not be dismissed lightly. Limited NHS resources, a reduction in GP registrars and specialist training for nurses makes the prospect of a GP/nurse partnership a viable option for the future.

Practice nurses can look forward to an exciting and challenging future.

Useful addresses

Department of Health
Richmond House
79 Whitehall
London SW1 2NL
www.dh.gov.uk

Medicines and Healthcare Products Regulatory Agency
www.mhra.gov.uk

National Prescribing Centre
www.npc.co.uk

Nursing and Midwifery Council
23 Portland Place
London W1B 1PZ
www.nmc-uk.org

Royal College of Nursing
www.rcn.org.uk

Working in partnership programme (Wipp)
www.wipp.nhs.uk
Supporting practices in resource management, and supporting practice nurses and healthcare assistants with learning packages and competencies.

References

Alcolado J (2000) Nurse practitioners and the future of general practitioners. *British Medical Journal* 320, 1084.
Ashby C (2006) The benefits of reflective practice. *Practice Nurse* 32(9), 35–37.
Bowles A (1995) Independent growth. *Practice Nurse* 8(12), 686, 688, 690–691.
Bradley E, Campbell P & Nolan P (2005) Nurse prescribers: who are they and how do they perceive their role? *Journal of Advanced Nursing* 51(5), 439–448.
British Medical Association (2004) *Quality Outcomes and Frameworks Guidelines.* www.bma.org.uk (accessed 28 June 2007).

Burns S (2006) Developing the health care assistant role. *Primary Health Care* 16(2), 21–25.

Carnwell R & Daly W (2003) Advanced nursing practitioners in primary care settings: an exploration of the developing roles. *Journal of Clinical Nursing* 12(5), 63–64.

Castledine G (1995) Defining specialist nursing. *British Journal of Nursing* 4(5), 264–265.

Chambers (2006) *The Chambers Dictionary 10th edn.* Edinburgh: Chambers Harrap.

Connechen J & Walter R (2006) Telephone triage in general practice. *Primary Health-care* 16(2), 36–40.

Cook R & Leech F (1996) Clinical supervision. *Primary Healthcare* 6(8), 12–13.

Cooper A (1997) Making skill mix work. *Practice Nurse* 13(9), 521–522.

Cross S (2006) Practice potential. *Nursing Standard* 20(43), 70–71.

Department of Health (1986) *Neighbourhood Nursing, A Focus for Care, Report of the Community Nursing Review.* London: HMSO.

Department of Health (1989) *DOH Report of the Advisory Group on Nurse Prescribing. The Crown Report.* London: HMSO.

Department of Health (1993) *The Challenges for Nursing and Midwifery in the 21st Century – a Report on the Heathrow Debate.* London: HMSO.

Department of Health (1996) *Choice and Opportunity. Primary Care: the Future.* London: The Stationery Office.

Department of Health (2000) *The NHS Plan.* London: Department of Health.

Department of Health (2002) *Liberating the Talents.* London: Department of Health.

Department of Health (2004) *Agenda for Change.* London: Department of Health.

Department of Health (2006a) *Improving Patients' Access to Medicines: a Guide to Implementing Nurse and Pharmacist Independent Prescribing Within the NHS in England.* www.dh.gov.uk

Department of Health (2006b) *Practice based Commissioning: Practical Implementation – What Does this Mean for Practices?* www.dh.gov.uk (accessed 12 January 2007)

Elton J & Bevan L (2005) Practice nurse performing minor surgery: the story. *Nursing in Practice* Mar/Apr, 67–69.

Fairfield H (1996) NVQ training in general practice. *Primary Health Care* 6(9), 14–16.

Fawcett Henesy A & West P (1995) Nurse practitioners: the South Thames Regional Authority experience. *Nursing Times* 91(12), 40–41.

Hopkins S, Hughes A & Vaughan P (2007) Healthcare assistants in general practice: delegation and accountability. *Primary Health Care* 17(1), supplement.

Learner S (2006) Prescription for Change. *Nursing Standard* 20(32), 20–21.

Lorentzon M & Hooker JC (2006) Nurse practitioners, practice nurses and nurse specialists: what's in a name? (30th Anniversary Editorial). *Journal of Advanced Nursing* 55(3), 273–275.

Macdonald JM (2005) Higher level practice in community nursing: part 1. *Nursing Standard* 20(9), 49–51.

Marsh GN & Dawes ML (1995) Establishing a minor illness nurse in a busy general practice. *British Medical Journal* 310, 778–780.

National Health Service Confederation/BMA (2003) *New GMS Contract. Investing in General Practice.* London: NHS Confederation/BMA.

National Health Service Executive (1996) *Clinical Supervision – A Resource Pack for Practice Nurses.* London: NHSE.

Nursing and Midwifery Council (2005) *Consultation on a Framework for the Standard for Post-Registration Nursing.* London: NMC.

Nursing and Midwifery Council (2006) *Standards of Proficiency for Nurse and Midwife Prescribers* London: NMC.

O'Dowd A (2006) New push for PBC. *Nursing Times* 102(49), 9.

Paniagua H (2001) *Practice made Perfect: Higher Level Aspirations for Practice Nurses.* London: Quay Books.

Parkinson C (1996) So you want to be a . . . GP practice partner. *Community Nurse* 2(4), 51.

Rashid A, Watts A, Lenehan C & Haslam D (1996) Skill-mix in primary care: sharing clinical workload and understanding professional roles. *British Journal of General Practice* 46(412), 639–640.

Reid J (2003) *Nurses Need to be All That They Can Be.* London: DH 2003/0462.

Richards DA, Meakins J, Tawfik J, Godfrey L, Dutton E, Richardson G & Russell D (2002) Nurse telephone triage for same day appointments in general practice: multiple interrupted time series trial of effect on workload and costs. *British Medical Journal* www.bmj.com/cgi/content.full/325/7374/1214 (accessed 21 January 2007).

Richards DA, Meakins J, Tawfik J, Godfrey L,Dutton E & Heywood P (2004) Quality monitoring of nurse telephone triage: pilot study. *Journal of Advanced Nursing* 47(5), 551–560.

Richardson G & Maynard A (1995) *Fewer Doctors? More Nurses? A Review of the Knowl-edgeBase of Doctor-Nurse Substitution.* York: The University of York.

Royal College of Nursing (1997a) *Practice Nursing and Skill Mix. Leaflet 42* London: RCN.

Royal College of Nursing (1997b) *Nurse Practitioners; Your Questions Answered.* London: RCN.

Royal College of Nursing (2004) *The Future Nurse: Evidence of the Impact of Registered Nurses.* www.rcn.org.uk/downloads/futurenurse/evidence-impact.doc (accessed 21 January 2007).

Royal College of Nursing (2005) *Nurses Employed by GPs. RCN Guidance on Good Employment Practice.* London: RCN.

Royal College of Nursing (2007a) *Employing healthcare assistants in general practice.* www2.rcn.org.uk/pcph/resources/a-z_of_resources/employing_health_care_assistants (accessed 21 January 2007).

Royal College of Nursing (2007b) *Administration of Medicines – Patient Group Direc-tions.* www2.rcn.org.uk/pcph/resources/a-z_of_resources/dminsitartion_of_medicine (accessed 21 January 2007).

Seale C (2006) Treatment advice in primary care: a comparative study of nurse practitioners and general practitioners. *Journal of Advanced Nursing* 54(5), 534–541.

Shum C, Humphreys A, Wheeler D, Cochrane M-A, Skoda S & Clement S (2000) Nurse management of patients with minor illnesses in general practice: multi-centre, randomised controlled trial. *British Medical Journal* 320, 1038–1043.

Smith M (1993) Skill mix in general practice. *Practice Nursing* 16 Nov-12 Dec, 21.

Stilwell B (1984) The nurse in practice. *Nursing Mirror* 158(21), 17–19.

Stilwell B (1988) The origins and development of the nurse practitioner. In A Bowling & B Stilwell (Eds) *The Nurse in Family Practice*. London: Scutari.

Stilwell B, Greenfield S, Drury M & Hull FM (1987) A nurse practitioner in general practice: working style and pattern of consultation. *Journal of the Royal College of General Practitioners* 37, 154–157.

The Information Centre (2007) *NHS Hospital and Community Health Services. Non-Medical Staff. England 199-2006*. www.ic.nhs.uk (accessed 14 May 2007).

United Kingdom Central Council (1993) *Final Report on the Future of Professional Education and Practice*. London: UKCC.

United Kingdom Central Council (1994a) *The Future of Professional Practice – the Council's Standards for Education and Practice following Registration*. London: UKCC.

United Kingdom Central Council (1994b) *Registrar's Letter 20*. London: UKCC.

United Kingdom Central Council (1996) *Registrar's Letter 15*. London: UKCC.

White M (2001) *Nurse Practitioners/Advanced Practice Nursing in the UK*. London: Royal College of Nursing.

Whitehead M (1988) *The Health Divide*. London: Penguin.

Wilson J & Bunnell T (2007) A review of the merits of the nurse practitioner. *Nursing Standard* 21(18), 35–40.

Index

The Informed Practice Nurse, Edwards, M. (2008), Chichester: Wiley.